The Pre-registration Interview

TOMORROW'S PHARMACIST

Welcome to *Tomorrow's Pharmacist* series – helping you with your future career in pharmacy.

Like the journal, book titles under this banner are specifically aimed at pre-registration trainees and pharmacy students to help them prepare for their future career. These books provide guidance on topics such as the interview and application process for the pre-registration year, the registration examination and future emplyment in a specific speciality.

The annual journal *Tomorrow's Pharmacist* will contain information and excerpts from the books in the series.

You can find more information on the journal at www.pjonline.com/tp

Titles in the series so far include:
The Pre-registration Interview: Preparation for the application process
Registration Exam Questions

The Pre-registration Interview

Preparation for the application process

Nadia Bukhari

BPharm, MRPharmS, PG Dip, PG Cert

Masters of Pharmacy Programme Manager
and Pre-registration Coordinator
School of Pharmacy, University of London, UK

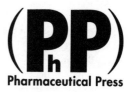

London • Chicago   **Pharmaceutical Press**

Published by the Pharmaceutical Press

An imprint of RPS Publishing

1 Lambeth High Street, London SE1 7JN, UK
100 South Atkinson Road, Suite 200, Grayslake, IL 60030-7820, USA

© Pharmaceutical Press 2007

(**PP**) is a trademark of RPS Publishing

RPS Publishing is the publishing organisation of the Royal Pharmaceutical Society
of Great Britain

First published 2007

Typeset by Photoprint Typesetters, Torquay, Devon
Printed in Great Britain by TJ International Ltd, Padstow, Cornwall

ISBN 978 0 85369 698 8

Disclaimer

The views expressed in this book are solely those of the author and do not
necessarily reflect the views or policies of the Royal Pharmaceutical Society of
Great Britain.

To my parents, whose efforts and encouragement
have made me the person I am today

Contents

Preface

Competition to acquire a position as a pre-registration pharmacist is currently at its peak. There are two principal factors contributing to this competition. First, there has been an increase in the number of pharmacy students graduating nationwide. Second, the number of posts available for newly graduated pharmacy students has remained stagnant. Therefore, it is paramount in this day and age to have that competitive edge to single oneself out from the rest of the crowd.

This book initially started as a collection of e-mails from fourth-year undergraduate students at the School of Pharmacy, University of London. The purpose of these e-mails was to provide feedback of students' interview experiences, which would be useful for the upcoming batch of students. Over the last 3 years, a vast amount of information has been collected and the best way to organise this information effectively is in a book format.

The information which students had given me was for the use of School of Pharmacy students only. As word spread, I started receiving e-mails from students nationwide asking for access to this material. This prompted me to go ahead and make this information available to all pharmacy students.

This book is intended to give students an insight into the application process for a pre-registration post. The questions in the question bank are real questions which students have had to tackle in an interview situation.

This is the first book of its kind and it is hoped that, with feedback from students nationwide, the information will increase, perhaps even showing up regional patterns.

Good luck and have fun applying!

Nadia Bukhari
February 2007

Acknowledgements

I wish to acknowledge the valuable support and input received from friends, students and colleagues at the School of Pharmacy, University of London.

I especially thank Ali Sameer Mallick for critically reading and editing selected portions of the book, providing constructive feedback and supplying a student's perspective.

I appreciate the help of Jiten Modha, Mandip Kudhail, Hassan Serghani, Mohammed Russell and Hashim Hashim for providing their CVs, application forms and covering letters, which were included in this book.

I thank the team at Pharmalife and Lloyds pharmacy, for allowing me to use their application forms, which will be invaluable for students.

I express my gratitude to the pre-registration team at Barts and the London NHS trust, Guys and St Thomas' NHS trust, Tesco and Astra Zeneca, for giving me the time to interview them.

I am extremely grateful to the Careers Service at the Careers Group, University of London, for permitting me to use sections of their careers leaflets on interview skills, application forms, covering letters and CVs. For further information on careers, visit their website at www.careers.lon.ac.uk.

I would like to express thanks to my editors at the Pharmaceutical Press, who have been very supportive, especially the senior commissioning editor, Christina De Bono, for her guidance and the development editor, Louise McIndoe.

Last, but not least, I wish to mention that without the support and encouragement of my loving husband, Murtaza Bukhari, this book could not have been possible – thanks a lot.

About the author

After qualifying, Nadia Bukhari worked as a pharmacy manager at Westbury Chemist, Streatham, London, for a year, after which she moved on to work for Barts and the London NHS trust as a clinical pharmacist in surgery. It was at this time that Nadia developed an interest in teaching, as part of her role involved being a teacher practitioner for the School of Pharmacy, University of London.

Two and a half years later, she began work for the School of Pharmacy, University of London, as the pre-registration co-ordinator for the school and the academic facilitator. This position involved teaching therapeutics to Masters of Pharmacy students and assisting the director of undergraduate studies.

Recently Nadia has taken on the role of the MPharm programme manager for the undergraduate degree.

Introduction

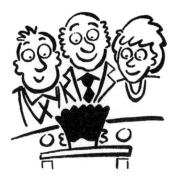

You are sitting in the waiting room, anticipating one of your most life-changing experiences to date. The room is unusually warm and you are accompanied by other applicants who are looking extremely pale. The atmosphere in the room is exceptionally tense. Your antiperspirant has just started to wear off and you start worrying about sweat patch marks on your shirt.

You decide to calm yourself down by drinking a glass of chilled water from a water cooler. However, you find it difficult to hold the glass steady. One of the other applicants glances at you and you nervously smile back. At that point, two people who could be mistaken for MI5 agents enter the room, and call out your name. You stand up and follow them as if they are taking you to your execution. Your time has come.

Interviews can be frightening experiences for a variety of reasons. First, there is an element of fear of the unknown. Human beings generally feel at ease when they know what to expect. Second, the stakes are extremely high. This interview could be the difference between a nice suburban house and claiming the dole! Finally, the confrontational nature of the interview is something nearly everyone dreads. Mix all these factors together, and you end up with a cauldron of distasteful broth.

This book cannot lower the stakes of the interview nor can it lessen the confrontational element. However, it can lessen the fear of the unknown by presenting valuable information supplied by students who have been in the same situation.

The intention of this book is to deal with students' ideas, concerns and expectations of the interview process. By addressing these three concepts, it is hoped that students will be more knowledgeable about the application process.

Tips are initially provided on how to apply for a pre-registration post and general interview technique. Then follows a vast selection of questions which students have faced in the past. With some of the questions, model answers have been provided. It is important to note that the purpose of these model answers is to stimulate your own thought processes rather than providing the ideal answer to a particular question. Remember, the key to success in answering any interview question is to give a unique answer.

In order to understand the ideas, concerns and expectations of students with regard to the interview process, fourth-year students at the School of Pharmacy, University of London, were interviewed. No doubt the sentiments they expressed are similar to those of other students.

Below are some quotations from students expressing their perceptions of the interview process.

IDEAS

What presumptions did you have about the interview?

'I thought you had to ask lots of questions but it was me doing most of the answering!'

'I thought I could manage my time effectively. However, trying to arrive on time for a big event is quite stressful.'

'I thought it would be as it was … but the interviewer was late!'

'I thought the panel would be old and mean. On the contrary, they were very welcoming and easy to talk to.'

'I knew it would be intense and it was. I knew it would be very competitive and I could sense that amongst the other candidates.'

'I thought the interview would be very knowledge-based. They asked questions on different areas of the undergraduate course, but there were more clinical questions. My community interview was more competencies-based.'

'I had presumed that I would get asked many clinical questions and views on white papers … and they came up!'

'I thought the interview would be very informal; I was wrong! It was very formal.'

'Hospital pharmacy interviews were more nerve-racking. I had more expectations as hospital pharmacy is very competitive.'

'I would say students should make themselves unique. I was quite nervous when I found out the interview would last 45 minutes. However, once I was in there, time flew by.'

'I knew questions about my degree and hobbies would come up, and they did!'

'We were expected to have much clinical knowledge. I had not prepared my therapeutics as I did not think they would ask much on it! Once I was in there time flew by.'

'I presumed that I would have a lot of clinical questions. They did not ask me anything clinical!'

'I anticipated questions on *Agenda for Change* and *Spoonful of Sugar* to come up; and guess what? They did!'

'I thought some panel members would be snobbish as competition is high. I thought smaller hospitals would be laid back but it's the same everywhere you go.'

'I expected the interviewers to be harsh but they were very friendly.'

Is there anything that would have helped you understand the process better?

'Not really. We had good support from university. We knew what to expect and the style of questions.'

'We had excellent preparation from university.'

'I would like to have had a clearer definition of prospects in community and hospital pharmacy and what kind of career progression is available.'

'We had a lot of guidance from university. I found it easy.'

'I had good support from our pre-registration co-ordinator.'

'The support from university was great! The interview question bank was invaluable.'

'I wish I had used the facility of having a pre-registration co-ordinator more as I felt I had no support from university.'

'I have a lot of work experience which helped me understand the process better, not to mention the support from university.'

'The question bank was very helpful. It built up my confidence.'

'I needed to get into grips with government papers. There is too much information and I just don't know how much we need to know.'

CONCERNS

What worried you about the interview most?

'Saying the right thing on the day and establishing a good relationship with the interviewers was a concern for me. I was very worried about getting clinical questions right.'

'Not getting the job was my biggest fear. I kept on making sure I was coherent and that I came across as competent.'

'The questions worried me the most. I wasn't sure if I was answering the questions how they wanted me to.'

'Clinical questions were a worry. I just had to prepare loads!'

'I hadn't had a placement related to pharmacy before so I needed to put in the extra effort to be more employable.'

'I had applied to a popular hospital so I was anxious about the competition.'

'I was nervous about whether I would know enough to get the job. The clinical questions were another worry and I just didn't know the calibre of them.'

'Clinical questions were a big concern. There are lots of drugs; which ones are they going to ask on?'

'I was nervous. I didn't know what to expect; having a **panel** of interviewers sounded daunting.'

'I was scared about being asked questions specific to a particular hospital where I haven't done a hospital placement. I was not sure what kind of clinical questions would be asked. I had no clue what the difference is between an inpatient and outpatient prescription.'

'Clinical questions and hospital-specific scenarios were causing me a lot of stress!'

'I just didn't know what to expect.'

'I was extremely nervous.'

'I was worried about being rejected.'

'Not being able to answer questions with confidence was a big worry for me.'

Is there anything that would have helped you prepare better?

'Having a mock interview would have been useful and having a question bank of interview questions would be very helpful.'

'It would have been beneficial if we had had more encouragement from our institution to read the *Pharmaceutical Journal* from the first year.'

'I wish I had done a hospital placement. It would have saved reading time on issues such as 'how do hospital pharmacists work' etc. I had to learn it all from scratch.'

'I think I was prepared for my interview. I would advise others to read what you have incorporated in your application form before you attend an interview.'

'I really wish I had done more reading on the future of the NHS and brushed up on the clinical-style questions.'

'I wish I had interview-style questions to prepare for my interview. A mock interview would be of great benefit.'

'I received lots of help. Our university gave a question bank to help us for the preparation of the interviews. I also talked to students from previous years on their experiences.'

'All hospitals were different from each other in terms of their approach.'

'I wish I had gone over more clinical issues rather than researching about the individual companies/hospitals, as I didn't need to go into too much detail at the interviews.'

'I had a dispensing test in an interview, which completely threw me!'

'I wish I had had a mock interview.'

'I should have done a hospital placement beforehand. It would have given me a better insight to the interview and the whole process.'

EXPECTATIONS

Was the interview experience as you expected? Why?

'Yes. I had prepared well and done the research. The structure was similar to what I had prepared.'

'Not really. I expected it to be more difficult and intense.'

'Yes. I expected it to be well organised and professional.'

'Yes. I had prepared for it well. Lots of structured questions were asked; not as many clinical questions were asked as I had thought.'

'They didn't ask as many clinical questions as anticipated.'

'It was better than expected!'

'It was friendlier than expected.'

'The interview was easier than expected. I had done a lot of preparation and everything had come up!'

'It was a relaxing and friendly atmosphere.'

'I had a surprise test (MCQs). Loads of clinical questions were asked. I was also given five prescriptions and had to analyse them.'

'It was easier than I had thought. Not as many clinical questions as I had thought. Most of the interview was about yourself.'

'Yes. I think they tested more than academic knowledge. I felt they pushed you on the day to see how much knowledge you have.'

'No. I found it very intimidating. No smiling! The panel were very hostile. I was expecting a barrier, but the set-up was informal. However, the interviewers were very scary.'

As you may gather, perceptions of the interview process vary from person to person. The process is also greatly dependent on where you are applying.

Before attending interviews, try and consult with students from former years who are currently doing their pre-registration at the hospital or company where you have applied. Another suggestion could be to visit the company/hospital of choice, where feasible. This will prepare you better for the big day and also remove the fear of the unknown, by giving you a brief insight on what to expect.

For the pre-registration year, students can apply to any of the three main sectors in pharmacy: hospital, community or industry. Over 90% of students apply for hospital and/or community pharmacy. Industrial placements for pre-registration students are limited. Not all companies participate in the programme, so it is worth contacting those drug companies that interest you to find out whether they do a placement or not. The companies that do offer a placement usually carry out a 50/50 split with either the hospital or community sector. It is advisable that students do not limit themselves by merely applying to one particular sector. The aim of the game is to have a pre-registration placement, so to increase your chances apply to all sectors. Once you have passed the examination, you can specialise in whichever sector you feel suits you best.

Summer placements

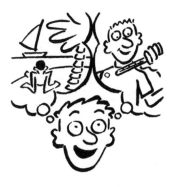

Have you thought what you will do once the summer vacation arrives? Most of you have probably booked a holiday or decided simply to laze about and enjoy the long 3½-month break.

Unfortunately, today's pharmacy student cannot afford to be so complacent. It is not suggested that you should not enjoy your vacations! Effective organisation of your time is recommended. Spend part of it in leisure and the rest carrying out summer placements. Working hard now will hopefully pay off when you apply for your pre-registration placements.

'I have another 2 years to worry about that!' most students would say. However in this day and age, when competition for a pre-registration place is getting tougher by the year, the summer vacations are the time for ambitious and determined students to carry out summer placements and increase their chances of obtaining the desired pre-registration placement in a couple of years. If you have experience in various pharmacy sectors, pre-registration employers will be more likely to invite you for an interview. You will be able to discuss your experiences at your interview, which will give you an upper hand over students without placements.

Every year approximately 2% of pharmacy students are unable to find a pre-registration placement. When asked what they might have done differently, they say that they wished that they had spent some of their vacation time doing placements!

It cannot be overemphasised how important it is to have experience of pharmacy in a practice setting. It gives you a chance to practise what you have learnt at university and to reinforce and build on transferable skills such as communication skills, time management and organisational skills.

WHY DO A PLACEMENT?

The number-one question: why should I waste my summer doing a placement? First, summer placements are great confidence builders, especially if you have no pharmacy experience. It helps you to develop skills and be more aware of issues involved in pharmacy.

Second, summer placements help academically. You should find it easier to retain drug names and understand when to prescribe certain drugs and when not to. When you return to university in the autumn term this will help you put theory into practice.

Third, doing summer placements in different sectors will make it easier for you to decide in which branch of pharmacy you want to work and apply for your pre-registration.

Fourth, when you do a placement well, employers remember you and will want to work with you again. If you apply to them for your pre-registration, they will remember you if you were a good worker and this will give you an advantage over other candidates.

Boots and Lloyds have started a new scheme: if you have successfully completed a third-year summer placement with them, they guarantee you an interview for pre-registration – you need not reapply. If you have been outstanding in your third-year summer placement some places may offer you a pre-registration place without an interview. It is anticipated that most large companies are now heading in this direction for their pre-registration recruitment.

HOW TO APPLY FOR A PLACEMENT

Applying for a summer placement is simple as long as you use your initiative. Most large companies and hospitals do a placement. The community applications are mostly online. You need to find out from individual companies when the application forms will be available for you to access. Some companies, such as Boots, hold road shows at universities where they give information on their summer placement schemes. So do try and attend these, as they are very informative.

If the industrial sector interests you, the best way of applying for a placement is by ringing round the various pharmaceutical companies and seeing which do a summer placement scheme. Not all companies do, so it is worth finding out. They will ask you to submit a CV and based on that they will invite you for an interview, after which they may or may not make you an offer. Some industrial companies have now started to visit universities and hold careers roadshows. If your university does not participate in this, ask them to contact the industrial sector.

If you are interested in doing a hospital placement, then you need to phone around the hospitals you are interested in to confirm whether they recruit summer-vacation students. Most hospitals will ask you to submit a CV with a covering letter and will give you a closing date for you application.

Some summer-vacation placements do offer a salary; however, some may not. They may offer to pay for your travel and lunch only.

It is appreciated that, for students, money is a huge incentive. However, even if it is without a salary and only for a month, it is nevertheless advised that you take on a summer placement. Remember: you reap as you sow. The benefits will become apparent later on when you apply for your pre-registration placement.

WHAT HAPPENS IN A PLACEMENT?

Placements vary from hospital to hospital and company to company. Their objectives, type of work and competencies are diverse. Hospital placements usually last 4 weeks whereas community and industrial placements usually last 8 weeks.

Below are examples of a summer placement programme in a renowned community pharmacy company, a well-known hospital and an eminent industrial company.

Community placement

For large companies, apply for a summer placement online. The form is similar to the pre-registration application form. Marks are given out of 40 for the entire application form; there are 5 marks for each question.

Students choose the location (area) where they wish to work; for example, London south or Surrey east. Students rank their areas and, depending on how well they score in the application form, they get their choice.

Currently, there is no interview for summer placements in large community pharmacy companies. This may change as competition rises.

Day 1 of placement

Vacation students have a regional induction with other vacation students working within the same company and region.

Here, pharmacy-related group activities are conducted. Students are confronted with scenarios and have to tackle them. For example, a customer comes to your pharmacy asking for a refund and is very angry. How would you deal with this situation?

Videos are then shown about the company, and on issues such as how to recognise counterfeit money and hazards in the workplace.

Day 2 and following

Students are introduced to the staff with whom they will be working and are given a tour of the store. Till training is carried out, preparing students to work over the counter.

Students work over the counter, advising customers as best they can and referring them to the pharmacist when necessary. They are expected to carry out a health care course during their placement. The course is theory-based, giving an explanation on each disorder and appropriate drugs to prescribe. Students are also expected to pass a calculation section in this course.

The course trains them on all the over-the-counter ailments and their treatments and prepares students on how to prescribe over-the-counter remedies and counsel patients. This demonstrates that this is a very valuable course to have completed.

Students also work in the dispensary towards the latter part of their placement. Here they are supervised and taught how to dispense medication correctly and efficiently. However, some pharmacies may not give students this opportunity. It depends on the pharmacist in charge and the store whether the student is allocated time in the dispensary. If the pharmacy is always busy, then it may be difficult for staff to train the student in the dispensary as they may have a pre-registration pharmacist who needs the attention more and is the priority.

Some pharmacies participate in the needle-exchange programme, methadone dispensing and the repeat prescription scheme. In the past summer-vacation students have been supervised and involved in these processes. If you are interested to participate in these schemes and have not already been offered, approach your pharmacist and explain your interest.

If you seem keen and interested, you will learn more and people will enjoy teaching you.

Assessment

A continuing professional development (CPD) file is given to you alongside a reflective diary which needs to be filled in daily and is marked weekly.

The tutor discusses the learning outcomes with students and keeps them on track with the health care course they are completing.

Hospital placement

Based on your CV you will either be invited for an informal interview or you may just receive an offer letter, depending on the hospital. If you are to have an informal interview, the questions asked are usually very basic. The interview is to help the employer find out a little bit about you and try and assess whether your personality would fit in their pharmacy environment.

Some examples of questions asked in previous summer placement interviews were:

- Why did you study pharmacy?
- What do you like about your course?
- Why do you want to do hospital pharmacy?
- What are your interests?
- What do you think is the role of the hospital pharmacist?
- Have you heard of *Agenda for Change*? What is it?

If you have completed a previous summer-vacation programme, they may talk to you about your experiences, which is a good thing as you can impress them with the skills you have achieved.

Reading the *Pharmaceutical Journal* regularly will help keep you up to date with recent pharmacy issues. So do access the site on a regular basis (www.pharmj.com).

The questions are very simple and straightforward – not as technical as the pre-registration interview!

Some hospital placements do not give students any dispensary work. Instead students carry out audits; for example, an audit on dispensary errors or waiting times in outpatient pharmacy. Alongside the audit, the student shadows ward pharmacists on their wards and receives some clinical exposure.

Other hospitals expose students to the dispensary from day 1 and they are usually dispensing during the entire placement. They also receive clinical exposure, by visiting various wards.

Some hospital placements do not offer clinical experience. If you are very determined to experience this, then you must approach your trainer or supervisor. If they observe your enthusiasm, they may set up a mini clinical programme for you.

Industrial placement

Again, based on your CV you will be invited for an informal interview or, if you are really lucky, get the placement without an interview.

Industrial placements are very interesting and challenging. If research and pharmaceutics are your forte, then this is the sector for you.

Day 1

This is usually an induction day when an introduction to the company is given and hazards, health and safety and, importantly, confidentiality are discussed. Company procedures and protocols are introduced.

Day 2 and following

Students are involved with clinical trials supply and packaging for the company. This includes:

- Labelling bottles. This is straightforward and a great way to get students familiar with their surroundings. As the title suggests, students simply label bottles to be used for clinical trials.
- Manufacturing clinical trials tablets. Students shadow other pharmacists or technicians and learn how to make tablets in the tableting rooms. Students then help with the tableting process by helping to set up powders. This would be supervised.
- Marketing for drugs on the market. Here students carry out research. For example, if the employing company produces an over-the-counter analgesic, the student researches to find out which drugs would be competitors to this drug. The research would include the benefits of the drug, comparing side-effects and clinical efficacy and, finally, how to make the drug more appealing to the public.
- Testing drugs. Students are also involved with testing drugs. For example, a powder is given to you and you have to discover what it is by finding out its solubility, pH and chemical properties. This information would help the company develop this powder into other formulations, such as intravenous injection.

It can be seen that industrial placements are very rewarding and students would have great exposure to the pharmaceutical world. This field is definitely one to consider.

If you do not get a formal summer placement in a large company or hospital, you can always try approaching the smaller independent pharmacies. It is better to have obtained some experience rather than none at all. Having a good experience at an independent pharmacy is just as valuable as having experience in a large chain. Your placement is what you make it. You could do a placement in a large company and not make the most of it, so you would not gain much. On the other hand, you could do your placement in a busy independent pharmacy and be involved with many services provided by the pharmacy, which will give you invaluable experience. So it is really your call.

SNIPPETS: IMPORTANCE OF SUMMER PLACEMENTS

Below are snippets from second- and third-year students at the School of Pharmacy, University of London, on their experiences and views on summer placements.

Why did you do a placement?

'I did a placement for experience and to have a good CV.'

'I wanted to improve my competency, build up confidence and improve clinical knowledge.'

'I wanted help with the pre-registration application process. I thought that if I do a placement, I will have a better chance of getting a pre-registration place.'

'I did it in order to have a range of experiences to help me with my pre-registration interview.'

'I wanted experience for the pre-registration year.'

'I did it to improve my chances of getting a summer placement in the third year.'

'I wanted more experience and help with the pre-registration year and interviews.'

How did you apply for a summer placement?

'Through university and road shows ... but also by using my initiative.'

'I went to a road show and applied from there. I asked employers what they were looking for.'

'Through friends ... if you know the right people.'

'I called up various companies and hospitals and e-mailed CVs everywhere. It didn't matter to me if the placement was paid or not, as long as I gained some experience.'

What did you gain from your placement?

'A good relationship with co-workers – they wanted me to come back!'

'Clinical knowledge: it helped to remember names of drugs.'

'It helped me to apply my knowledge.'

'I did my dispensing validation, which helped with pharmacy practice at university.'

'It broadened my horizons in the pharmacy world.'

'It helps to talk about past experiences in interviews – a good icebreaker!'

'I feel I am more confident. My communication skills have improved immensely; I felt I could handle responsibilities. I really felt mature.'

'I have a much better understanding of pharmacy. I can feel the transition before and after.'

'My communication skills have improved and I have a better insight to pharmacy.'

Did the placement meet your expectations?

'It was a lot harder than I thought. I felt like giving up at times, but it was worth the hard work.'

Hospital: 'Shadowing the pharmacist helped me increase my knowledge.'

Community: 'Health care assistant's course had a structured programme, and was invaluable as it can be used anywhere.'

'Yes, and more. Boots had good training! The training was structured, and there were meetings with a tutor.'

'The placement was excellent. It exceeded my expectations and I feel I have grown in this placement.'

'All the students I was working with really enjoyed the placement and thought it was better than expected.'

What advice would you give someone thinking of doing a placement?

'Do it! It is a great confidence builder, you gain a lot of experience and it looks good on your CV.'

'Apply to as many places you can; present yourself well on paper. Ask friends for advice and make sure you know the new developments in pharmacy.'

'Do one! There is a lot of competition. Do one from your first year. Leaving it to your third year is too late.'

'Do it early, as it's hard to get a placement in the third year.'

'Do it, because it stands you in very good stead. You gain more experience, and you are more likely to get your chosen placement. It is very competitive.'

'Do as much as you can so you know what you are going in for.'

'Do one! It gives you experience and you feel like you know something once you have done one.'

'Do it; even if it means travelling, do it. It helps with pre-reg and during your course.'

'Start applying in your first year. Don't be afraid to apply. It is tough to get a pre-reg placement, so the more experience you have, the better.'

A summer placement is what you make it. If you show enthusiasm and initiative, you may learn and experience more than your colleagues. So it really is up to you what you learn and how much exposure you receive in your placement.

Applying from your first year is sensible; you can never have enough experience. Obtaining a summer placement is very competitive; do not be afraid to travel. The placement is only for a short time and the exposure will be of value to you. As mentioned previously, you reap as you sow.

Good luck and remember: use your time effectively!

Where and how to apply

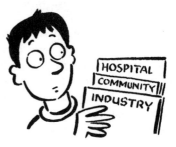

HOW TO APPLY

This chapter will provide a quick summary of how to apply for your pre-registration placements. If you have been through the summer placement application process, you will already be familiar with some of this.

Every pre-registration site in the UK is listed in the document called the *Royal Pharmaceutical Society of Great Britain (RPSGB) Approved Premises for Pre-registration Training.* You can access this document through the RPSGB website (www.rpsgb.org/members/preregtraining/index.html). Scroll down to Approved Pre-registration Premises and click on the link that says 'click here'. You can search for approved premises by town or postcode and by the type of place you want – community, hospital or industry.

For independent pharmacies, you must apply directly to the various pharmacies, as they do not usually send universities information or application forms. You should apply by sending a CV and covering letter.

Community

Most community groups (e.g. Boots, Moss, Lloyds) hold a road show, either at your university or at an outside venue. They talk about their pre-registration programme and distribute application forms if they are still using them. Many now have online applications so they may talk you through how to complete these online. Closing dates are usually around the end of June or July of each year.

Boots does not recruit pre-registration pharmacists unless they have completed a third-year summer placement programme with them. If Boots is one of your choices, then you must ensure that you apply for a summer placement programme with them. As mentioned before, most large companies are moving towards this initiative for their recruiting.

For most organisations interviews are held at the end of August or early in the autumn term of the fourth year of study. Previously, some organisations even offered positions on the same day as the interview!

The organisations that do not visit the universities usually send their application packs directly to each university and students can collect these from their careers department. The large multiples will usually have application forms or online recruitment, but when you deal with some of the smaller chains or with independent pharmacies, you may have to provide a CV with a covering letter in lieu of an application form.

During and after company presentations, you should ask questions and talk to the representatives. They want to get to know you. The more inquisitive you are, the more likely they are to remember you. It is also in your interest to find out as much as you can about their pre-registration programme so that you can make an informed decision about whether you wish to apply to a particular company.

Dates for each company's presentations should be provided by your careers department. If you do not have a careers department, then you may be able to find this information on the companies' websites, or simply by ringing them at the beginning of the academic year when you are in your third year of the MPharm programme.

Hospital

For pre-reg places in NHS hospitals in England and Wales, there is a clearing house system like UCAS called Pharmalife. Around mid-March, universities receive information packs which include a thick booklet with a brief description of each hospital offering pre-registration places. These packs may be picked up from your university careers department. NHS Scotland recruits separately and you will find information on this as well as Northern Ireland and Eire at the end of this chapter.

The closing date for applications is the end of August at the end of your third year of study, so you have ample time to make your choices. The forms are to be filled via the online application form. Here, you include your preferred hospital sites. You have to provide name and address details for two referees so that the clearing house can contact your two referees by e-mail. One point to note: always ask for permission before you put a name down as a referee. It is both polite and professional to do so. Failure to do so may spoil you receiving a decent reference. However, as the literature will explain to you, the submission of referee details has to be done earlier than the closing date, to allow time for the referees to be chased. The interview dates vary from hospital to hospital, often depending on the popularity of the hospital. Most interview in mid to late September. By early October, students know whether they have secured a place or not. Students living overseas should think about returning to the UK slightly earlier than usual to avoid missing any interviews.

If you do not receive an offer of a place, there is a second round, or the clearing of applications, when hospitals with unfilled vacancies readvertise. You can reapply by early November. Interviews are quick and posts are offered by mid-November.

The website with the online application is usually not ready for use until March or April, and this is usually after the pre-reg booklet has been produced and sent to pharmacy schools. This booklet contains details of all the hospitals offering pre-reg places. There are descriptions of the hospitals and the code numbers you need to use when you choose your hospitals on the online application form.

If you are looking for hospital pre-reg places, ask your careers office to show you the literature on other NHS regions.

There is nothing to stop you contacting any hospital to make preliminary enquires about the places they will advertise in the main recruitment booklet in April/May. You may, for example, want to know if a hospital can provide you with accommodation, or you may want to know whether the hospital specialises in a particular field.

If you are interested in the NHS north-west region, which covers hospitals in Liverpool, Manchester, Bolton, Burnley and Blackpool, there is an excellent website at: www.doh.gov.uk/nwro.nwpharm.

Split placements with industry

Every year some students enquire about split industrial placements. These are usually linked with a hospital placement. A booklet called *RPSGB Approved Premises for Pre-registration Training* gives you information on which companies offer these split placements.

Interviews and offers

Most interviews are held in mid-August to early September. Some employers like to interview early, others slightly later. The *RPSGB Guidance for Pre-reg Employers* states that students should not be pressurised into accepting offers and gives a date, which varies from year to year (see Appendix 1). To check the latest guidance, see the RPSGB website (www.rpsgb.org.uk).

Such guidance gives students the chance to attend more than one interview before making a final decision. If an employer is pressurising you for a reply before the set date given in the guidance, you should inform the Pre-registration Division at the RPSGB, as explained in the guidance.

WHAT TO DO NOW?

Three things you should think about now are:

- Referees
- Preparing your CV and cover letter
- Finding a summer work placement for the end of your third year, especially if you did not have one the previous summer

First you need to think about who would be a suitable referee. Every application form will ask for at least one referee, usually two, so you should think about those members of staff who know you well. This may be your academic tutor, your project supervisor or someone else who has taught you. My advice is that your first referee should be an academic and the second referee a pharmacy employer (or another employer if you have not yet worked in a pharmacy). You must ask permission first before you put anyone's name on an application form.

It cannot be overemphasised how important it is to have work experience in a pharmacy during the course. Pre-reg employers look for this and students who do not have such experience on their CV are at a distinct disadvantage. See the chapter on summer placements for further information.

NHS Northern Ireland, NHS Scotland and Eire

If you are interested in doing your pre-reg in Scotland, Northern Ireland or the Republic of Ireland, contact the careers department at your university. For places in Scotland, the application procedure is similar to that in England and Wales. Your university should receive a CD-ROM pack which lists all the hospitals in Scotland offering places. It is an online application procedure.

The Pre-Reg Handbook

Universities should receive copies of *The Pre-registration Handbook* from the RPSGB. Most universities distribute this to students; some have it in their careers department. This magazine contains numerous articles on pharmacy and life after graduation. There are also several pages of adverts, mainly from community organisations, as well as some from individual NHS trusts or regions. This is a very informative read, so make sure you get hold of a copy!

WHERE TO APPLY

Whether you are interested in specialising in hospital, community or industry, it is recommended that you apply everywhere. Places are limited and competition is high. Once you have completed your pre-registration training and qualified as a registered pharmacist, you can apply for jobs in the sector on which you wish to focus.

Competition is rising and it is getting hard to secure a pre-registration place. Do not limit yourself further by only applying for placements near your university town or home. Although many students wish to live at home and commute to work, you are further narrowing your chances by limiting yourself to pre-registration places in a specified area.

London in particular is very competitive and most large teaching hospitals and many branches of large chains are there. However, in England there are many other counties with hospitals and branches of the large community companies and industrial companies, offering a pre-registration placement. It would be wise to apply out of London to increase your chances of getting a place. Remember: it's not where you do your placement, it's what you make of it.

Many students who wish to work in London still apply in London but also choose to apply outside London to increase their probability of getting a pre-registration placement. What you should bear in mind is that it is only for a year, and even if you have to live away from home, it may be quite an experience for you. I cannot stress enough that you should not limit your applications and stay confined to one particular area.

For some students, salary plays a significant role, as students' loans need to be paid and other personal commitments take precedence. However, there is not too much difference in salary between each sector. Nevertheless, there are competitive salaries within each sector. For example, one community company might offer a couple of thousand more per annum than its competitor.

Below is a rough estimate of salaries per annum in 2006 in each pharmacy sector:

- Hospital: £17 000–£23 000
- Community: £15 000–£18 000
- Industry: £20 000–£24 000

Third-year undergraduate students at the School of Pharmacy, University of London, were asked questions on what they felt was important to them about the pre-registration year.

SNIPPETS: WHAT IS IMPORTANT TO STUDENTS ABOUT THE PRE-REGISTRATION YEAR?

What is important for you about the pre-registration year?

'I want to be comfortable with the job I am in. I want to be learning new things, developing my skills, and having experience with patients. Salary is not really that important to me. I just want to get a place and pass the year.'

'I want to gain experience and practise as a pharmacist in real life. I want to be learning more and putting things I learnt at university into context.'

'This will be a transition from student to professional for me.'

'I want to be prepared for it. I have a lot of expectations. I want to gain confidence as a pharmacist. I'm not sure if my expectations will be met, though.'

'I just want to get a placement. It doesn't matter where. It's getting hard to get placements so I just want to get one anywhere.'

'I want to learn as much as possible and get good training.'

'Passing! I want to pass the registration exam. I want to be able to get enough experience so that I can work as a pharmacist on my own. I hope I have a good tutor to guide me.'

'I want to have the confidence to work as a pharmacist on my own.'

'Passing the exams is top of my list!'

'I want to be able to experience what being a pharmacist is like in real life and how to run a business and learn the practicalities of the pharmacy.'

'I want to build confidence in medicines and diseases so I have more experience when advising my patients. I want to attain the skills of responsibility, time management and the ability to multitask.'

How would you select where you want to do your pre-registration placement?

'It would help if I did my placement with a big company, as it is better known, more respected, and other employers would know the place I have trained from. I would want the company to have good training to help me pass the exams.'

'I would want to apply to the big teaching hospitals. I have spoken to students who have worked in teaching hospitals, and they tell me that you gain more experience there as you have good tutor support and structured learning. If you are working in London then salary is important, as the cost of living is higher.'

'Money is not a factor for me. I just want a place, anywhere!'

'I would wish to go to a large teaching hospital, as they are well known and have a good reputation. It would also help me when I finish my pre-reg year when I am looking for a job. I do want a decent salary and I have been told that London has better salaries. I would also like to look at applying to a specialist hospital in London.'

'I just want a pre-reg place so that I can pass the exams. I think you need to be motivated by yourself; it doesn't matter where you go. You should make the most of your placement.'

'I want to be near home, somewhere local, somewhere where the competition is less. I would want to do my placement in a large company as training will be good. Salary is not important for me.'

'To choose my place I will talk to my friends in the year above, visit employers' websites, and visit locations. Having good training is important for me. Salary is not important. I just want get through the year.'

'I wish had done more placements so you know what you are going in for. I will apply to places where I have done a placement and go to road shows. I think I will apply everywhere.'

'Money is not a factor as it is a training year. Having a good tutor is important. I will be mature about this and not confine myself to London. I am looking for an established programme of training, and a well-known, reputable company. I would prefer to work in a busy pharmacy as you are likely to learn more.'

'The hospital's reputation is important. I would also ask other students who have done a pre-reg placement at the hospital how the training is. Salary doesn't matter to me.'

Do you have any apprehensions about the pre-registration year/process?

'Not really. I'm not sure how much experience to have.'

'Not really. I am worried about not getting a place and what to do if I don't get one.'

'If I don't get a placement then I would not want to reapply. I may go for a career change.'

'No. I am looking forward to working as a pharmacist.'

'There is a lot of competition. I just want to know how to be certain of getting a place!'

'Yes. I am not sure if I have enough experience. I fear that I may be rejected.'

Do you have any concerns about the pre-registration application process?

'I don't know if I will have enough experience. How can I stand out above the others? Interviews worry me and presenting yourself on the day is a big worry. Finally, will I even get a place?'

'I am scared of doing interviews; I get nervous. I have never had an interview before. I can't think on the spot.'

'Interviews are my biggest worry. If I have a large panel interviewing me, I may feel intimidated and nervous. Once I get past the first question hopefully I will calm down and everything will flow naturally. The exam is already worrying me – having the burden of three attempts to do it.'

'I just want to know what employers are looking for. I am not sure if I have enough experience. Interviews sound daunting. I don't know what employers expect and what kind of questions they will ask me.'

'The lack of experience in interviews is my main concern.'

'I am scared of interviews. I don't know what is expected. I find some application forms hard to fill in; I just don't know what they want me to say.'

'I hate the application form questions. I really don't know how to answer them. What can you say that is different from others? It's all so scary!'

'Interviews are my biggest fear! I haven't done one before – there is fear of the unknown. I don't know how you are meant to act on the day, and what you do if you are asked an awkward question. I just want a job!'

'Yes: I hate the application forms. I just don't know what to write and I feel like I am being arrogant as I am just selling myself. I don't know what they are expecting.'

'Yes. I am extremely worried about the interview. I don't know how to act in interviews. I feel that it's not a fair indicator of my personality.'

'I prefer having an interview. I am just worried about the application forms as they are very wordy and technical.'

Students from other schools of pharmacy will probably share similar fears and views as the School of Pharmacy students. It is anticipated that most of these concerns will be addressed in this book.

Students' biggest fears are interviews. The chapter How to Conduct Yourself on the Day and the sample questions will help students be better equipped for the big day.

The chapter on The Application Process will give students a better insight of what the applications forms look like and give advice on how to fill them out.

The application process

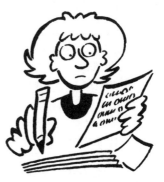

The application process for the pre-registration year is very demanding. There are three stages:

- Stage 1: deciding where to apply (see chapter on Where to Apply)
- Stage 2: applying via application forms/CV
- Stage 3: interview

Most companies have an online application process; some may ask you to submit a CV with a covering letter; others may ask you to complete an application form.

In this chapter, some handy tips on CV and application form-writing will be given.

Also incorporated in this chapter are example application forms from Lloyds Pharmacy and Pharmalife (hospital pharmacy). This will train students and give an insight to the application process.

CURRICULUM VITAE

Your CV is a selling tool. It sells you and your qualities to a prospective employer. Therefore, it is important that you offer and express yourself in the best way that you can.

The beauty of a CV is that you can include as little or as much as you like about yourself – you are in control of its content. This will allow you to develop a powerful marketing tool which is tailored around yourself.

You should also include points that you would like prospective employers to discuss with you at the interview.

It should be appreciated that employers receive thousands of CVs for one job and it is quite mundane for them to read through each one and make decisions. Employers usually decide whether the CV is a good or bad one in the first 5 seconds! So you need to make your CV attractive, short and easy to read (the layout should be clear).

It is very easy to put your whole life story in the CV, but that is not what is required! Short relevant points will be of benefit and easy for the employer to read.

Most CVs have the following six sections:

- Personal details
- Education
- Work history
- Skills
- Interests and activities
- Referees

Personal details

These usually consist of your:

- Name
- Address (with relevant dates, if you have a term-time and home address)
- Telephone number
- E-mail address

Note: Supplying information about your age, nationality and gender is optional.

Education

List:

- Details of your university education
- A levels (or equivalent) with grades

Rather than writing out all your GCSEs (or equivalent), note how many you attained. However, if certain GCSEs are required for the job you wish to apply for, then list the details for these specific qualifications.

If the work you are applying for will make direct use of your subject, give full details of your degree – for example, an overview of the degree as a whole, a list of relevant courses you took or a description of a final-year project or other important feature.

Work history

There are various ways you could list the jobs you have done:

- Reverse-date order (the most recent first)
- To save repetition, you could divide your work experience into categories according to relevance to the job or industry, such as: 'media-related' and 'additional'
- You could group similar jobs together, even if they happened at different times, summarising the skills you gained

Employers are often interested in all the work experience you have had (paid and voluntary), particularly if it shows you have general qualities that they value, such as the ability to work in a team, lead a team, be in charge of a project, meet deadlines, work under pressure and take responsibility. Consider mentioning exactly what it was about the jobs you did that developed skills such as these, and do not just list the tasks you carried out in your different jobs.

Skills

Employers are often interested in specific skills you have acquired, such as:

- foreign languages
- computing languages or packages

Try to give specific details, for example about your level of proficiency in foreign languages, degree of familiarity with computer packages and so on.

You might choose to include other relevant transferable skills in this section, such as communication, teamwork and organisation. This works well when you have developed that skill in various ways, e.g. from your education, interests and work experience, and want to avoid repeating yourself in each section of your CV. It is also particularly helpful to focus on skills gained if your previous work experience bears little obvious relation to the job for which you are now applying.

Interests and activities

You could include:

- leisure activities and interests, e.g. sports, music, cultural activities
- membership of clubs and societies
- positions of responsibility
- travel

Do not just list your interests. Show how they have developed qualities the employer will value.

Referees

CVs are usually two pages long, so include full references if you want to or are asked to, but if you run out of space it is perfectly acceptable to write 'Reference available on request'.

It is very important that you have a good CV and often it is hard to make a start on it. Examples of two CVs are shown in Figures 1 and 2. One is a CV which, in my opinion, is to a high standard, and the other requires much improvement. Having a look at both CVs will ignite ideas for your own CV. It is easy to copy a fellow peer's CV; however, the employer will figure out within minutes that it is not your own CV from the language you use at the interview. Individualise your CV: it is **your** CV, so keep it that way! The CVs provided in this book are inspiring, and it will be to your disadvantage if you decide to copy them verbatim.

Figure 1 Example of a bad CV.

CURRICULUM VITAE

Correct personal details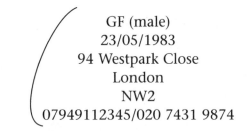

GF (male)
23/05/1983
94 Westpark Close
London
NW2
07949112345/020 7431 9874

Personal Statement

Very -> colloquial

Avoid abbreviations

My punctuality and attendance are excellent, and in my experience, this is what many employers have problems with. As I have worked in retail for 2 years, I have excellent communication skills with customers, where I always offer the best possible advice and help to customers. I am an experienced sales person/assistant with strong selling abilities. I am till-trained and can work as a cashier. I'm able to work with others in a team and can follow instructions at all times. As a person, I'm organised, hard-working, determined, polite, confident, aspirational and very respectful. I possess key skills in communication, number and IT that equip me in a working environment.

Education and Qualifications

- I'm currently studying Pharmacy at **The School of Pharmacy** (University of London). I have successfully passed the first 2 years, and am at present well into the first semester of my third year, which I started in October 2006.

Secondary education/sixth form – Hampstead Comprehensive School. Dates: 1996 – 2003

- A/AS Levels – 3 A levels and 1 AS level were sat in the summer of 2003: Chemistry – A, Biology – B, Electronics – C, Maths – D
- GCSE's – 9 subjects were sat in the summer of 2001: English Literature – A, English language – A, Maths – A, Science – BB, French – B, Physical Education – A, History – C, Design technology – C
- I have a Key Skills qualification in communication

Figure 1 *continued*

- I have a HSBC certificate of achievement in cashiering.
- I have a junior sports leader award.

Employment History

- Recently, June 2005, I worked for 1 month in a community pharmacy known as **Craig Thompson Chemist**. There I was able to gain vital experience in dealing with every day issues that a pharmacist is faced with, like dispensing and offering patient advice, and general shop work, I thoroughly enjoyed the experience.
- In the summer of 2002, I worked at **Royal Free Hospital** where I was able to converse with patients in the wards, talk to them about there illness'. I dealt with patient records and patient history. I also worked on the clinical desk, and I also did some administration work in the office.
- I just finished working at **JJB Sports plc**; I've was working there for the past two years, where I was a sales assistant. My work involves interacting with customers, selling trainers to customers, stock room/delivery work and general retail work around the store.
- Recently, I did some temporary work in the stock room of **Zara**. My work involved organising, tagging and the pricing of clothes.
- In the summer of 2001, I worked in **Willesden Sports Centre** for a month, where I did some life-guarding, admin work and general leisure assistant work.

Not laid out well. Employers' details should be stated clearly, as headings, with the job description underneath

Aspirations

No focus in the field of pharmacy

Hopefully, in a few years' time I would like to become a practising pharmacist in a hospital or a community pharmacy, and would also like to play semiprofessional football as a part-time career.

Expand and explain

Interests

Football, travelling, reading, films, music, dancing and culture.

References

No skills section. Has this student sold himself as well as he could?

Available on request.

Surname?

William – Assisstant manager at JJB sports: call him on 020 8208 2155 for a reference.

Figure 2 Example of a good CV.

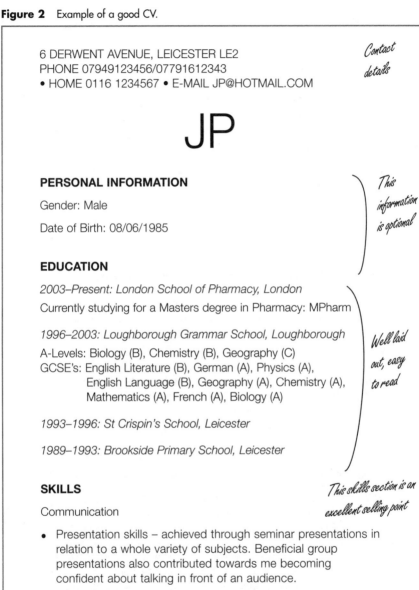

6 DERWENT AVENUE, LEICESTER LE2
PHONE 07949123456/07791612343
• HOME 0116 1234567 • E-MAIL JP@HOTMAIL.COM

Contact details

JP

PERSONAL INFORMATION

Gender: Male

Date of Birth: 08/06/1985

This information is optional

EDUCATION

2003–Present: London School of Pharmacy, London
Currently studying for a Masters degree in Pharmacy: MPharm

1996–2003: Loughborough Grammar School, Loughborough
A-Levels: Biology (B), Chemistry (B), Geography (C)
GCSE's: English Literature (B), German (A), Physics (A),
    English Language (B), Geography (A), Chemistry (A),
    Mathematics (A), French (A), Biology (A)

1993–1996: St Crispin's School, Leicester

1989–1993: Brookside Primary School, Leicester

Well laid out, easy to read

SKILLS

Communication

This skills section is an excellent selling point

- Presentation skills – achieved through seminar presentations in relation to a whole variety of subjects. Beneficial group presentations also contributed towards me becoming confident about talking in front of an audience.
- Customer liaison – as a grocery assistant I was communicating with a wide range of customers, answering queries and complaints, which helped develop my interpersonal skills.
- Sales skills – comprehending the product knowledge allowed me to assess customer needs by advising them to take different approaches in order to find certain products.

Figure 2   *continued*

Teamwork

- Group presentation required time management, co-operation and motivating each other to achieve successful outcomes.
- Being a platoon leader in the army division in CCF enabled me to take charge and lead in an effective manner to ensure that our tasks were fulfilled.

Creativity

- Fluent in Gujarati and English as well as strong conversational French, German and Italian.
- Computer-literate in word-processing, spreadsheets and statistical packages.

EMPLOYMENT HISTORY

22 June 2002–16 August 2004: Asda Oadby, Leicester: Availability/grocery colleague. Responsibilities included dealing with customer issues both effectively and efficiently in order to maintain a high level of customer satisfaction. Duties included effective control with the continual rotation of stock and replenishment, adjusting counts, space-flexing and price-changing.

June 2001–December 2002: Aigburth Methodist Homes for the Aged, Leicester: Domestic cleaner. Responsible for the general cleanliness and tidiness of the care home, whilst maintaining a high standard of cleanliness. This was my first experience in a full working environment.

This student has subcategorised his work experience

PHARMACY EXPERIENCE   *between pharmacy and non-pharmacy related*

31 August 2006–26 August 2006: Boots Summer Placement Programme, Dorset: A 4-week summer placement, which continued from my previous year's experience. New aspects included attending medication usage reviews (MURs), patient group directions in hair retention and weight loss. Conducted patient care plans, which enabled me to understand the importance of MURs, whilst enabling me to become more familiar with the newer services Boots offer.

3 July 2006–28 July 2006: Whittington Hospital, Archway, London:
Concise job description. Good use of language
A 1-month placement carried out in both an inpatient and outpatient dispensary. Shadowed pharmacists on a variety of wards and vastly improved my clinical knowledge. Also attended the warfarin clinic and worked in medicines information. This

Figure 2 *continued*

placement, in a much larger hospital, confirmed for me that my aspiration lies in hospital pharmacy and validated my decision to carry out hospital pre-registration placement.

2 March 2006–10 June: Erasmus Programme, Milan, Italy: For a 12-week period I carried out a laboratory-based research project at the University of Milan. My research area was focused on the cardiovascular effects of sildenafil and I gained a valuable insight into the necessity for research. The cultural experience was also thoroughly enjoyed. Whilst in Italy I also gained a level 1 diploma in Italian.

17 August 2004–Present: Asda Pharmacy, Oadby, Leicester: Pharmacy assistant. Responsibilities included helping and serving patients with over-the-counter medicines, dispensing prescriptions as well as counselling patients when required. Blood pressure checks were also carried out in accordance with the new pharmacy contract. General clerical duties and stock control were essential parts of the job.

3 October 2005–Present: British Pharmaceutical Student Association (BPSA) Representative: Currently the BPSA representative for the London School of Pharmacy. The BPSA is a branch of the Royal Pharmaceutical Society of Great Britain, which represents all pharmacy undergraduates and pre-registration students. Responsibilities include organising conferences, activities and events at the university as well as providing students with pharmacy-related news and information. *This*

27 June 2005–26 August 2005: Boots Summer Placement Programme, Dorset: This 2-month placement was unique as the store was located in a very busy doctor's surgery. During my time here I gained more clinical knowledge, through shadowing a doctor, a cardiac and a gastro specialist nurse. Responsibilities included dispensary duties and assisting customers with over-the-counter medicines. New aspects that I encountered included the procedures involved in dispensing methadone and Ministry of Defence prescriptions. Whilst here I also passed my health care assistant's course and gained an insight into the business aspect of the company.

student has had a lot of work experience and has really sold himself

24 March 2005: Responding to Symptoms Patient Counselling Competition, Nottingham: The purpose of this competition is to measure students' ability to acquire information needed to provide the correct treatment, as well as the ability to communicate information. In this competition I reached the UK finals, which were held at the BPSA Annual Conference in Nottingham, where I represented my university.

Figure 2   *continued*

19 July 2004–13 August 2004: Bassetlaw District General
Hospital, Worksop: Pharmacy assistant. A 4-week voluntary
placement which was carried out in a busy dispensary. The
pharmacy services comprised a busy inpatient and outpatient
dispensary, clinical ward rounds and a sterile production suite. My
responsibilities included dispensing both inpatient and outpatient
prescriptions and assisting on the clinical ward rounds, whilst
shadowing the pharmacist. During my time here I gained my
dispensing validation and a valuable insight into hospital
pharmacy and thoroughly enjoyed the clinical experience.

Work Experience June 2001: Sam's Chemist, Glen Parva: This
work experience was carried out in a large independent
pharmacy. Duties included assisting with sales of over-the-counter
medicines, stock control and observing the prescription process.
Outcomes included learning the importance of strong teamwork,
communication skills and general administrative skills.

Original interests, clearly stated.

INTERESTS AND ACTIVITIES

I have played for the second eleven in hockey for my school as well
as attending the gym on a regular basis, which indicate my passion
to keep fit and live a healthy lifestyle. I also study the martial art of tae
kwon do, which enables me to maintain my fitness levels. In my spare
time I enjoy reading and listening to music as well as socialising with
friends.

This student really stands out

REFERENCES

NB   Mrs. KP
Pre-registration Tutor   Bassetlaw District General
The School of Pharmacy   Pharmacy Department
                                        Worksop
                                        Nottinghamshire SB1 0BD
                                        Tel: 1234567

There are three other examples of CVs in Appendix 2. The CVs included in this appendix have a mixture of good and bad points. It has been left to you to analyse which are the good and which the bad tips.

COVERING LETTERS

The covering letter is the prerequisite to your CV. If your covering letter is impressive, the employer will then take a glance at your CV. So you need to take time and care when constructing your covering letter.

Introduction

This first paragraph needs to be very clear: include who you are (recently graduated with a 2:1 Masters of Pharmacy from the University of Bath), why you are writing (to apply for *x* position; looking for work experience) and where you saw the position advertised or, if it is a speculative application, where you heard about the organization.

Why have you applied to that particular company?

Use this section to tell employers why you want this particular job with their particular organisation; this is your chance to impress them with your commitment and enthusiasm. Demonstrate that you understand what the job involves and that you have researched their company. Avoid vague statements and blatant flattery; be specific and illustrate your opinions with some original points.

Why should they employ you?

Now is your chance to impress on the employer why you are just right for this job, in terms of skills, experience and personal attributes. Illustrate your unique selling points with three or four excellent examples, rather than trying to cover everything. Use the organisation's recruitment information to guide you towards the particular skills and competencies that they want and highlight your evidence of them.

Highlight your specific strengths, motivations and reasons for applying. Convey a confident, competent, enthusiastic and professional attitude. Avoid any spelling, grammatical or typing errors. Ask a friend to check your letter before you post it.

Covering letters are also an opportunity to explain in a positive way any gaps or apparent weaknesses in your CV, such as poor academic results due to illness, for example.

Greetings

Always try to find a name, rather than a job title, as it demonstrates to the employer that you have done your homework and have researched the organisation. Dear Ms Smith is much better than Dear Sir/Madam.

Take time when writing your closing paragraph, as it is an important opportunity both to restate your interest and to summarise your suitability for the post. It is also a good place to state your availability for interview and to end on an optimistic and polite note.

Examples of covering letters are shown below. One lacks professionalism (Figure 3) whereas the other is to a very high standard (Figure 4). (More examples can be found in Appendix 2.)

Figure 3 Example of a bad covering letter.

Dear Catrin Thomas ———→ *This should be Ms/Mrs/Miss Thomas*

Hi, my name is HP, I'm 20 years old and I am currently a *Very colloquial, informal language*
Pharmacy student at the School of Pharmacy, University
of London. I am well into the first semester of the third
year of the MPharm course which I started on October
4 2005.

I am very interested in obtaining a place within the *Poor English*
summer placement programme within your hospital
pharmacy organisation.

I wish to apply for summer placement at your hospital as I
understand that it's a busy district general hospital
providing a complete range of clinical services. There is a
large orthopaedic department and one of the largest day-
surgery units in the country and the hospital has a
specialist eye unit which has its own casualty department,
which is all impressive. The pharmacy department must be
very demanding as they provide pharmaceutical services
to other hospices.

I feel that it is important to gain experience within a
hospital pharmacy as it is coming close to my pre-
registration year, so it will give me a better chance of
obtaining a desired place.

Clinical pharmacy is a challenging, varied and
rewarding profession and one which I would like to be a
part of. I would like to fulfil a variety of medicines-related
functions, such as performing clinical duties on wards or
in outpatient clinics and being involved in the day-to-day
dispensing of medications, which may include formulary

Generally, a badly written covering letter, with poor use of language. The student has undersold himself. In today's highly competitive environment, this letter would probably be rejected

Figure 3 *continued*

management and the promotion of cost-effective prescribing. Hospital pharmacists routinely have access to the list of drugs that patients are currently prescribed in hospital, In order to provide the best possible advice to the patient, I want to experience working closely with the doctors as part of the multidisciplinary team for patient care. Also in the London School of Pharmacy we have been taught specialist activities, for example, the aseptic assembly of sterile pharmaceuticals (such as reconstituting antibiotic injections) which I understand are not taught in other pharmacy schools.

My background in community pharmacy should make me suitable for this position. At the beginning of the summer holidays (June/July), I worked in a community pharmacy in Willesden Green for about a month; the pharmacy was called Craig Thompson Chemist; he is a very nice chap. I was covering for his dispenser who went on holiday. My work involved obtaining the prescription from the patient, dispensing the medicine required, having the pharmacist do the final check and finally giving the medicines advice to the patient, and dealing with over-the-counter and P medicines. Also CD register updating, handling CDs, counselling and dealing with computer systems. My work also involved dealing with deliveries and orders, sorting out prescriptions, stock management, ensuring dispensary is organised and tidy, deliveries, operating tills, cashing up, attending to customer services and some basic shop work. I thoroughly enjoyed the experience.

Closing paragraph not very convincing

During my placement I wish to acquire skills needed to be a competent pharmacist.

I have enclosed a copy of my CV.

Thank you   *Student has not signed off*

Figure 4 Example of a good covering letter.

64 Derwent Avenue
Leicester
9 February 2007

Pharmacy Department

Dear Mrs X

I am writing with regard to the prospect of any paid or unpaid work experience within the pharmacy department at X Hospital. Enclosed is a copy of my CV.

I am currently a third-year undergraduate on the MPharm degree at the London School of Pharmacy. I would like to put in writing my keen interest to be considered for an opportunity that might arise during the coming summer vacation between the following dates: 19 June–29 September 2007. I fully appreciate that it may not be possible for a position for much of this period, but I would like to state my willingness to consider whatever you may have to offer me.

Sound language

Working in a hospital pharmacy would be the perfect opportunity to gain an invaluable insight into the role of a hospital pharmacist. As I have already carried out a voluntary work placement during my first year at Doncaster Bassetlaw Hospital I would very much appreciate it if I could gain a further insight into what I personally believe will be my future career. My aim is to build on everything that I have learnt during my studies and see the theory being put into practice. One of my areas of interest is cardiology and I believe myself to be very patient and highly responsible and I have a great willingness to listen and learn – these are just some of the many key strengths I have to offer.

Carefully thought out and beautifully laid out

Figure 4 *continued*

My skills also include being able to communicate very well with others, being a strong team player and a hard worker with an ever-enthusiastic and positive approach. I am a self-motivated and well-organised individual with a committed approach to my work. If unfortunately nothing is available this coming summer, I would appreciate being put forward for a placement in the summer of 2008.

Finally, I would like to take this opportunity to thank you for considering my application. I would be very pleased to come for an interview where I can expand on my CV.

Thanking you in advance

Good closing paragraph

Sincerely,

JP   *Appropriately signed off*

APPLICATION FORMS

Application forms require more consideration than the CV. Much planning is involved so do not rush. Questions can be quite specific or vague, thus thinking about each answer logically before writing and submitting the application form is recommended. Some students fill out their application form 2 or 3 days before the deadline, having been unable to judge how time-consuming it really is. An outstanding application form guarantees an interview. This is something that involves perseverance and dedication.

Handy hints for filling in application forms

- Read it through carefully and note any specific instructions. If they ask you to write in block capitals or black ink, do just that.
- Tailor your answers to what you have discovered about the job and the kind of person best suited to fill it.
- Draft answers in rough first. It may help to take a photocopy of the form so that you can work on the layout of your answers.
- Think about why an employer may be asking this question. What do they want to know?
- If a question is not applicable, say so. Do not leave empty boxes.
- Use positive and specific words to describe your activities and interests, rather than vague terms and tired clichés.
- Check for spelling mistakes and grammatical errors before writing the final version (and after!).
- Avoid beginning sentences with I.
- Use different examples for different questions.
- Stick to word limits.
- If you have to hand-write the form, make sure that it is legible.
- Always keep a copy of the form so that you can remember what you wrote.
- Keep an eye on the closing dates.

Decide what you want the answer to achieve

It is worth working out first, on a separate piece of paper, precisely what you want to achieve with your answer.

Organise the evidence

Work on a separate piece of paper. You might:

- assemble the facts that support your answer
- choose the evidence that seems to be most appropriate
- think out how you can use the chosen material

Stick to the word count

If the main points you have decided to make are of equal weight, you could then use your chosen material to produce three equally weighted paragraphs (1. Describe the issue, 2. how did you solve it? 3. What was the conclusion?). Remember to use positive and specific words.

Edit the three paragraphs down to about 250 words

You will almost certainly need to revise the draft to ensure that it hangs together as a whole, relates appropriately to other answers on the form and will fit comfortably in the space provided.

Copy the final draft on to the form

When you are satisfied with the answer, write on the form itself, taking great care to achieve a high standard of presentation.

An example of a student's application form is shown in Figure 5. This student took much time and effort when filling in his application form and it is very well written. This application form gave him many job interviews and he managed to secure a pre-registration placement without any problems.

Figure 5 Example of an application form.

> **Tell us why you chose pharmacy and why you want to work in hospital pharmacy.**
>
> My desire to work with people in an area of science where there is still much to be discovered is what attracted me to pharmacy. I have chosen pharmacy as a prescription for a rewarding future as it has many career pathways with the flexibility to change and the opportunity to meet people from all walks of life.
>
> Before choosing what career path to follow, I undertook placements in a wide region of the health sector. I preferred pharmacy because pharmacists are the final contact of patients with the health system in most cases, which forms a path for educating patients on the use of their medications.
>
> The bottom line is that pharmacists help patients get well, which unquestionably makes it a rewarding and satisfying profession. Hospital pharmacists play a major role in the health care team, giving advice and expertise on treatment regimens and issues across clinical practice, and this is what drew me to pharmacy. From personal experience hospital pharmacists are better prepared, more skilful and more experienced in clinical pharmacy.
>
> I aspire to achieve a career in hospital pharmacy as I am intrigued by the increasingly important role of the pharmacist. I am also very intrigued by the idea of direct involvement with patient care provided by hospital pharmacy.
>
> Hospital pharmacy offers a structured career pathway allowing me to train and then specialise, providing me with a wide and varied career and allowing me to study for further academic qualifications.

Figure 5 *continued*

Tell us about your social and recreational interests.

I am an amateur photographer with special interests in stills and portrait pictures. I undertook self-directed learning to further my knowledge and techniques in photography. I am currently learning about digital picture editing.

I thoroughly enjoy travelling as it has allowed me to understand and experience different cultures. I recently travelled to Dubai, United Arab Emirates and Bahrain. I was able to travel around these countries and have the opportunity to speak to local people to gain a better understanding of their history and culture. I used my photographic skills to capture some of the great scenic views and local people.

Sport plays an important role in my life, especially football. I played for a local club for 3 years, reaching the top three teams in 2 consecutive years. Football has also enabled me to improve my communication skills with my colleagues. Currently I have also started to play badminton.

Reading journals such as *Hospital Pharmacist* and *Pharmaceutical Journal* frequently, I am kept up to date with the current issues pharmacists are facing and different changes coming into effect. This allows me to develop my own perspective on the issues and how pharmacists are affected.

Add anything else you want to tell us.

From my extensive work placement history, both pharmacy- and non-pharmacy-related, I have gained various different skills. Some of the skills I have gained from my work placements are listed below:

Figure 5 *continued*

Management

Precise, accurate delegation of tasks to all members of staff is a key skill that I have developed and enhanced throughout my experiences, which has enabled me to deliver an excellent quality of service.

Communication

I have gained excellent verbal and non-verbal communication skills through working as a pharmacist in the community, counselling patients, negotiating with other professionals and giving clear instructions to members of staff.

Teamwork

I have developed highly motivated team-working skills by working in many fields that require a high degree of teamwork, primarily as a pharmacist with members of staff, ensuring the pharmacy runs effectively.

Problem-solving

Through my experiences as a pharmacist assistant, I have developed systematic diagnostic problem-solving skills to find precise solutions to problems, ensuring the satisfaction of all parties.

IT/computing

I am computer-literate in several packages such as Word, Excel and PowerPoint. I have been able to use these skills for assignments where interpretation of data is necessary, and in researching articles on the internet.

It cannot be overemphasised how important your CV and application forms are when applying for a pre-registration place. They are the gateway to the interview, and then you have the chance to sell yourself in person and make a lasting impression.

Time, care and attention are required when completing these. As mentioned before, do not start filling out your application forms shortly before the deadline. Give yourself at least 2 weeks before the deadline to have completed the forms, as this allows you to think carefully about what you are writing. If you spend time and effort on your application forms and CVs, employers will see that you have done so. It is easy to spot an application that has been rushed.

The next few pages show screen shots of the application forms provided by Lloyds and Pharmalife (Figures 6–13). This will give you a taster of how an application form for pre-registration appears and also prepare you, so you can evaluate how much work it entails.

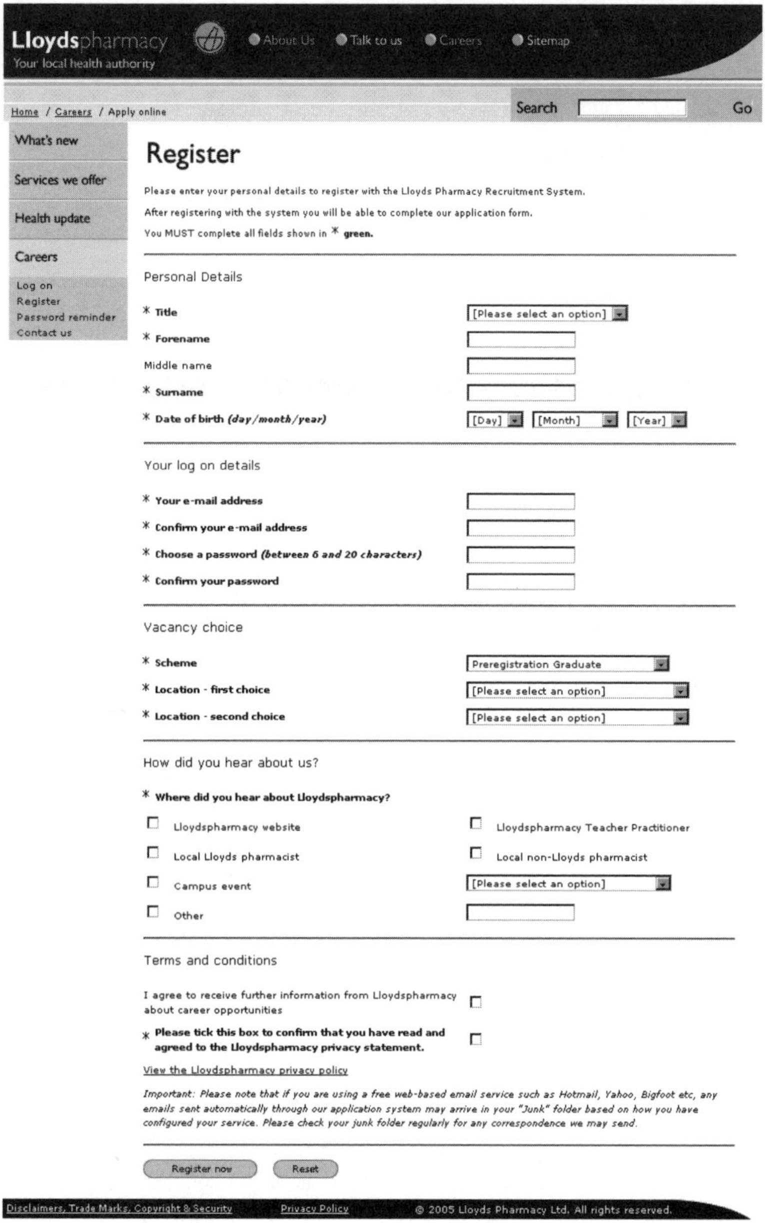

Lloydspharmacy
Your local health authority
About Us | Talk to us | Careers | Sitemap

Home / Careers / Apply online
Search [ ] Go

What's new
Services we offer
Health update
Careers
Log on
Register
Password reminder
Contact us

Register

Please enter your personal details to register with the Lloyds Pharmacy Recruitment System.
After registering with the system you will be able to complete our application form.
You MUST complete all fields shown in * **green.**

Personal Details

* **Title** [Please select an option]
* **Forename**
Middle name
* **Surname**
* **Date of birth** ***(day/month/year)*** [Day] [Month] [Year]

Your log on details

* **Your e-mail address**
* **Confirm your e-mail address**
* **Choose a password** ***(between 6 and 20 characters)***
* **Confirm your password**

Vacancy choice

* **Scheme** Preregistration Graduate
* **Location - first choice** [Please select an option]
* **Location - second choice** [Please select an option]

How did you hear about us?

* **Where did you hear about Lloydspharmacy?**

☐ Lloydspharmacy website
☐ Lloydspharmacy Teacher Practitioner
☐ Local Lloyds pharmacist
☐ Local non-Lloyds pharmacist
☐ Campus event [Please select an option]
☐ Other

Terms and conditions

I agree to receive further information from Lloydspharmacy about career opportunities ☐

* **Please tick this box to confirm that you have read and agreed to the Lloydspharmacy privacy statement.** ☐

View the Lloydspharmacy privacy policy

Important: Please note that if you are using a free web-based email service such as Hotmail, Yahoo, Bigfoot etc, any emails sent automatically through our application system may arrive in your "Junk" folder based on how you have configured your service. Please check your junk folder regularly for any correspondence we may send.

Register now | Reset

Disclaimers, Trade Marks, Copyright & Security | Privacy Policy | © 2005 Lloyds Pharmacy Ltd. All rights reserved.

Figure 6 Lloyds registration page. This is where you submit your personal details in order to register on their site. All online application forms have a registration page. (Reproduced with permission.)

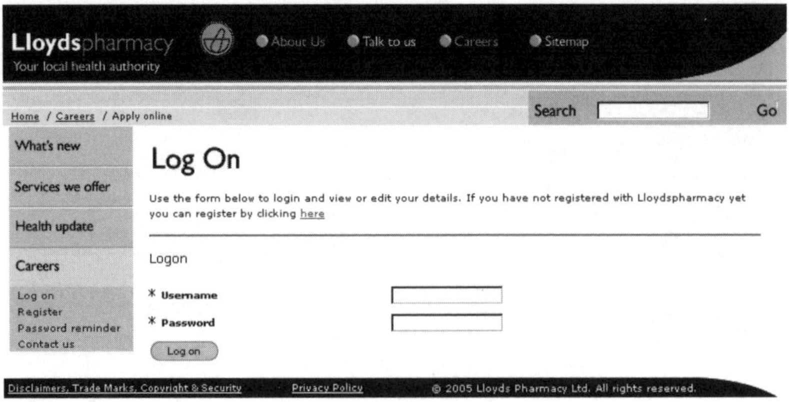

Figure 7 You then log on with the user name and password, which you provided when you registered on the site. (Reproduced with permission.)

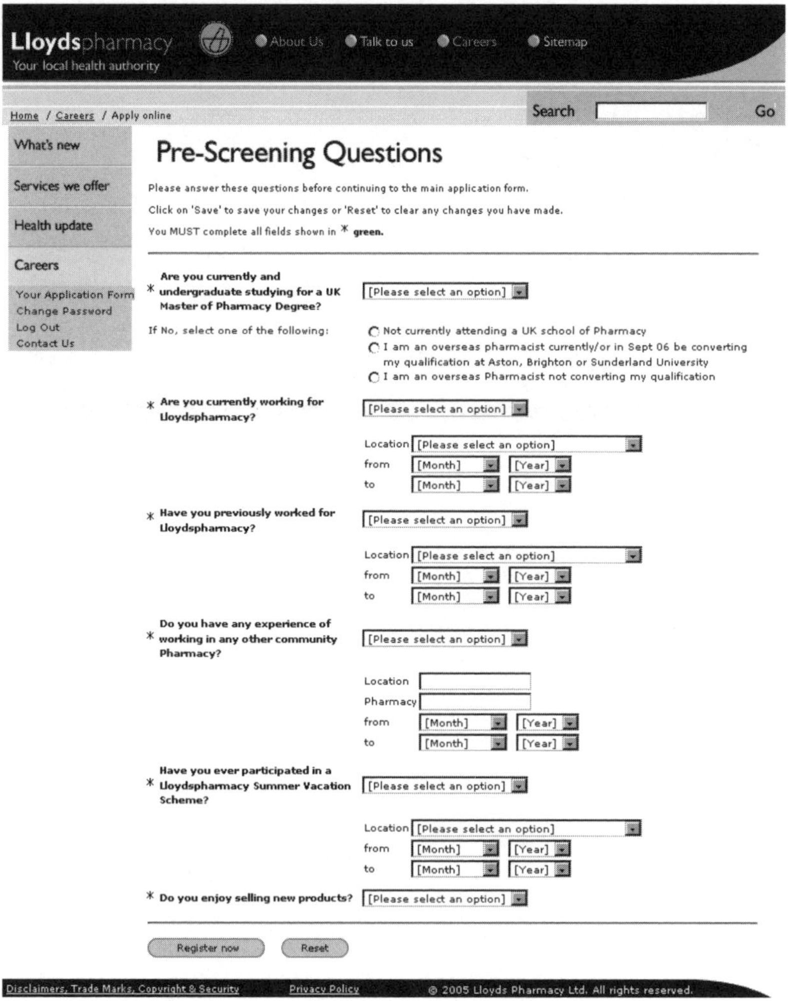

Lloydspharmacy
Your local health authority

About Us · Talk to us · Careers · Sitemap

Home / Careers / Apply online

Search [ ] Go

What's new
Services we offer
Health update
Careers
Your Application Form
Change Password
Log Out
Contact Us

Pre-Screening Questions

Please answer these questions before continuing to the main application form.

Click on 'Save' to save your changes or 'Reset' to clear any changes you have made.

You MUST complete all fields shown in * **green.**

* **Are you currently and undergraduate studying for a UK Master of Pharmacy Degree?** [Please select an option]

If No, select one of the following:
- Not currently attending a UK school of Pharmacy
- I am an overseas pharmacist currently/or in Sept 06 be converting my qualification at Aston, Brighton or Sunderland University
- I am an overseas Pharmacist not converting my qualification

* **Are you currently working for Lloydspharmacy?** [Please select an option]

Location [Please select an option]
from [Month] [Year]
to [Month] [Year]

* **Have you previously worked for Lloydspharmacy?** [Please select an option]

Location [Please select an option]
from [Month] [Year]
to [Month] [Year]

* **Do you have any experience of working in any other community Pharmacy?** [Please select an option]

Location
Pharmacy
from [Month] [Year]
to [Month] [Year]

* **Have you ever participated in a Lloydspharmacy Summer Vacation Scheme?** [Please select an option]

Location [Please select an option]
from [Month] [Year]
to [Month] [Year]

* **Do you enjoy selling new products?** [Please select an option]

Register now · Reset

Disclaimers, Trade Marks, Copyright & Security · Privacy Policy · © 2005 Lloyds Pharmacy Ltd. All rights reserved.

Figure 8 These are pre-screening questions which need to be filled in before you complete the application form. Read these questions carefully so that you are clear what is being asked of you. (Reproduced with permission.)

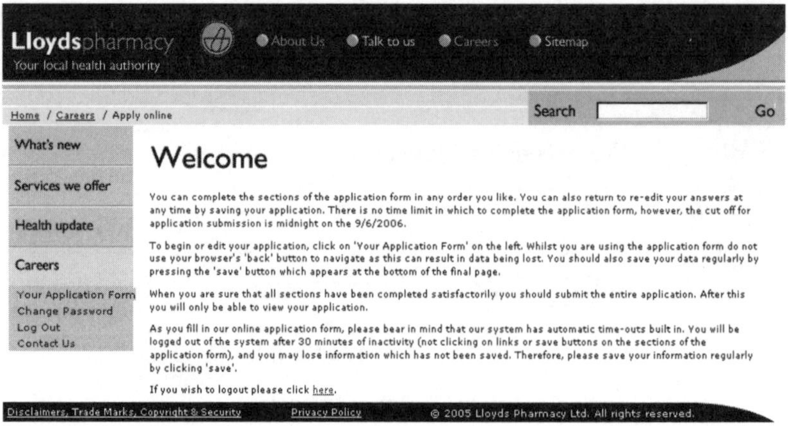

Figure 9 You are now through to the application form pages. (Reproduced with permission.)

Figure 10 *(opposite)* Your personal details need to be completed. Ensure that you provide an accurate address and contact number. Provide your mobile number as well as your landline. This will allow prospective employers to contact you easily. (Reproduced with permission.)

Lloydspharmacy
Your local health authority

● About Us ● Talk to us ● Careers ● Sitemap

Home / Careers / Apply online

Search [   ] Go

What's new

Services we offer

Health update

Careers

Your Application Form
Change Password
Log Out
Contact Us

Personal Details

On this page you can add to, view and change the information you have provided about your personal details.

Click on 'save' to save your changes or 'reset' to clear any changes you have made.

* Title	[Please select an option] ▾
* Forename	[ ]
Middle name	[ ]
* Surname	[ ]
* Date of birth *(day/month/year)*	[Day] ▾ [Month] ▾ [Year] ▾
* E-mail address	[ ]
* Correspondence Address Line 1	[ ]
Correspondence Address Line 2	[ ]
* Correspondence Address Town	[ ]
Correspondence Address Region	[ ]
* Correspondence Address Postcode	[ ]
* Correspondence Address Country	United Kingdom ▾
Correspondence Address Other Country	[ ]
Term-time Address Line 1	[ ]
Term-time Address Line 2	[ ]
Term-time Address Town	[ ]
Term-time Address Region	[ ]
Term-time Address Postcode	[ ]
Term-time Address Country	[Please select an option] ▾
Term-time Address Other Country	[ ]
* Contact Number	
Contact Number Day	[ ]
Contact Number Evening	[ ]
Contact Number Mobile	[ ]
* Do you hold a current UK driving licence?	○ Yes ⦿ No
* Are you eligible to live and work in the UK?	○ Yes ⦿ No
If no please give details	[ ]
* Nationality	[Please select an option] ▾
Do you have any criminal convictions? [Declaration subject to * Rehabilitation of Offenders Act - convictions defined as spent under the Rehabilitation of Offenders Act should not be mentioned.]	⦿ Yes ○ No
* Gender	[Please select an option] ▾
* Ethnicity	[Please select an option] ▾
If other please specify	[ ]
* Do you have a disability?	[Please select an option] ▾
If other please specify	[ ]

(Next) (Reset)

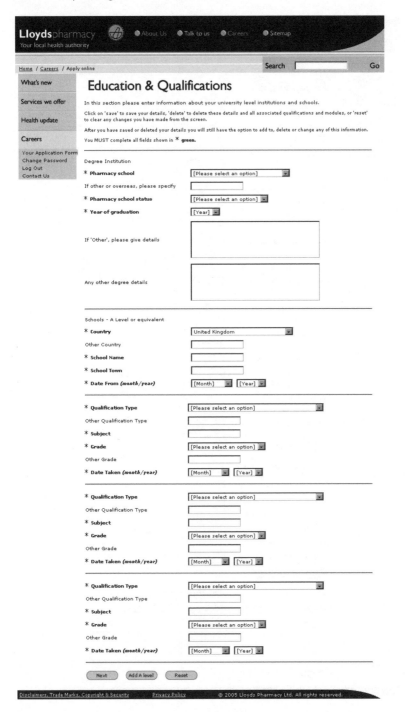

Lloydspharmacy
Your local health authority

● About Us   ● Talk to us   ● Careers   ● Sitemap

Home / Careers / Apply online

Search [   ]   Go

What's new

Services we offer

Health update

Careers

Your Application Form
Change Password
Log Out
Contact Us

Education & Qualifications

In this section please enter information about your university level institutions and schools.

Click on 'save' to save your details, 'delete' to delete these details and all associated qualifications and modules, or 'reset' to clear any changes you have made from the screen.

After you have saved or deleted your details you will still have the option to add to, delete or change any of this information.

You MUST complete all fields shown in ✱ **green.**

Degree Institution

✱ **Pharmacy school**   [Please select an option] ▼

If other or overseas, please specify   [   ]

✱ **Pharmacy school status**   [Please select an option] ▼

✱ **Year of graduation**   [Year] ▼

If 'Other', please give details

Any other degree details

Schools - A Level or equivalent

✱ **Country**   United Kingdom ▼

Other Country   [   ]

✱ **School Name**   [   ]

✱ **School Town**   [   ]

✱ **Date From** *(month/year)*   [Month] ▼ [Year] ▼

✱ **Qualification Type**   [Please select an option] ▼

Other Qualification Type   [   ]

✱ **Subject**   [   ]

✱ **Grade**   [Please select an option] ▼

Other Grade   [   ]

✱ **Date Taken** *(month/year)*   [Month] ▼ [Year] ▼

✱ **Qualification Type**   [Please select an option] ▼

Other Qualification Type   [   ]

✱ **Subject**   [   ]

✱ **Grade**   [Please select an option] ▼

Other Grade   [   ]

✱ **Date Taken** *(month/year)*   [Month] ▼ [Year] ▼

✱ **Qualification Type**   [Please select an option] ▼

Other Qualification Type   [   ]

✱ **Subject**   [   ]

✱ **Grade**   [Please select an option] ▼

Other Grade   [   ]

✱ **Date Taken** *(month/year)*   [Month] ▼ [Year] ▼

(Next)   (Add A level)   (Reset)

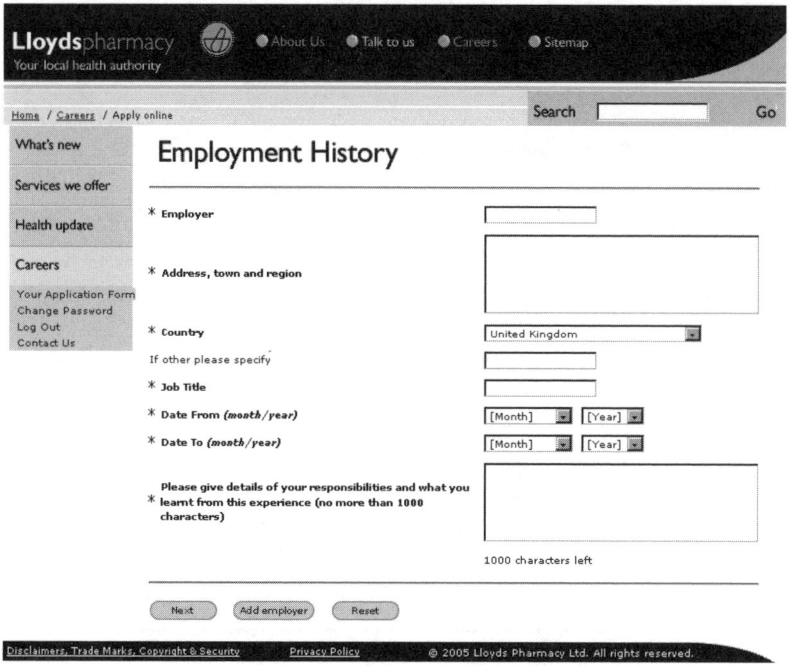

Lloydspharmacy
Your local health authority

● About Us ● Talk to us ● Careers ● Sitemap

Home / Careers / Apply online

Search [　　　　　　] Go

What's new

Services we offer

Health update

Careers

Your Application Form
Change Password
Log Out
Contact Us

Employment History

* **Employer** [　　　　　　　]

* **Address, town and region** [　　　　　　　]

* **Country** [United Kingdom ▾]

If other please specify [　　　　　　　]

* **Job Title** [　　　　　　　]

* **Date From** *(month/year)* [Month ▾] [Year ▾]

* **Date To** *(month/year)* [Month ▾] [Year ▾]

* **Please give details of your responsibilities and what you learnt from this experience (no more than 1000 characters)** [　　　　　　　]

1000 characters left

(Next) (Add employer) (Reset)

Disclaimers, Trade Marks, Copyright & Security　　　Privacy Policy　　　© 2005 Lloyds Pharmacy Ltd. All rights reserved.

Figure 11 *(opposite)* This page is similar to the education section of a CV. Here you need to provide information of your academic history. (Reproduced with permission.)

Figure 12 This is the employment history page. If you have had more than one employer, you can add this by clicking the 'Add employer' button. When giving details of your responsibilities, write them out first on a piece of paper, modify and check the details, and then type this online. Double-check for any spelling and grammatical errors. (Reproduced with permission.)

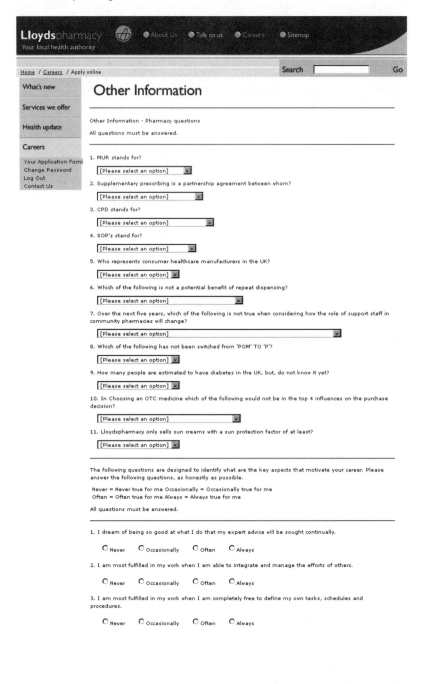

Lloydspharmacy
Your local health authority

● About Us ● Talk to us ● Careers ● Sitemap

Home / Careers / Apply online

Search [   ] Go

What's new

Services we offer

Health update

Careers

Your Application Form
Change Password
Log Out
Contact Us

Other Information

Other Information - Pharmacy questions

All questions must be answered.

1. MUR stands for?

[Please select an option] ▼

2. Supplementary prescribing is a partnership agreement between whom?

[Please select an option] ▼

3. CPD stands for?

[Please select an option] ▼

4. SOP's stand for?

[Please select an option] ▼

5. Who represents consumer healthcare manufacturers in the UK?

[Please select an option] ▼

6. Which of the following is not a potential benefit of repeat dispensing?

[Please select an option] ▼

7. Over the next five years, which of the following is not true when considering how the role of support staff in community pharmacies will change?

[Please select an option] ▼

8. Which of the following has not been switched from 'POM' TO 'P'?

[Please select an option] ▼

9. How many people are estimated to have diabetes in the UK, but, do not know it yet?

[Please select an option] ▼

10. In Choosing an OTC medicine which of the following would not be in the top 4 influences on the purchase decision?

[Please select an option] ▼

11. Lloydspharmacy only sells sun creams with a sun protection factor of at least?

[Please select an option] ▼

The following questions are designed to identify what are the key aspects that motivate your career. Please answer the following questions, as honestly as possible.

Never = Never true for me   Occasionally = Occasionally true for me
Often = Often true for me   Always = Always true for me

All questions must be answered.

1. I dream of being so good at what I do that my expert advice will be sought continually.

○ Never   ○ Occasionally   ○ Often   ○ Always

2. I am most fulfilled in my work when I am able to integrate and manage the efforts of others.

○ Never   ○ Occasionally   ○ Often   ○ Always

3. I am most fulfilled in my work when I am completely free to define my own tasks, schedules and procedures.

○ Never   ○ Occasionally   ○ Often   ○ Always

4. Security and stability are more important to me than freedom and autonomy.

   ○ Never   ○ Occasionally   ○ Often   ○ Always

5. I am always on the lookout for ideas that would permit me to start my own enterprise.

   ○ Never   ○ Occasionally   ○ Often   ○ Always

6. I will feel successful in my career only if I have a feeling of having made a real contribution to society

   ○ Never   ○ Occasionally   ○ Often   ○ Always

7. I will feel successful in my career only if I face and overcome very difficult challenges.

   ○ Never   ○ Occasionally   ○ Often   ○ Always

8. I dream of a career that will permit me to integrate my personal, family and work needs.

   ○ Never   ○ Occasionally   ○ Often   ○ Always

9. I will feel successful in my career only if I can develop my technical or functional skills to a very high level of competence.

   ○ Never   ○ Occasionally   ○ Often   ○ Always

10. I dream of being in charge of a complex organisation and making decisions that affect many people.

   ○ Never   ○ Occasionally   ○ Often   ○ Always

11. I would rather leave my organisation, than accept an assignment that would undermine my ability to be of service to others.

   ○ Never   ○ Occasionally   ○ Often   ○ Always

12. I dream of having a career that will allow me to feel a sense of security and stability.

   ○ Never   ○ Occasionally   ○ Often   ○ Always

13. Building my own business is more important to me than achieving a high level managerial position in someone else's organisation.

   ○ Never   ○ Occasionally   ○ Often   ○ Always

14. I am most fulfilled in my career when I have been able to us my talents in the service of others.

   ○ Never   ○ Occasionally   ○ Often   ○ Always

15. I see out work opportunities that strongly challenge my problem solving and/or competitive skills.

   ○ Never   ○ Occasionally   ○ Often   ○ Always

16. Balancing the demands of personal and professional life is more important to me than achieving a high level managerial position.

   ○ Never   ○ Occasionally   ○ Often   ○ Always

17. Please select the TWO statements from 1-16 which MOST apply to you

Statement 1 that most applies is   [Please select an option] ▼

Statement 2 that most applies is   [Please select an option] ▼

(Save) (Reset) (Submit Application)

Figure 13 This is the final page. The first section comprises 11 pharmacy-related questions. If you are unsure of any of the answers, look them up – don't guess! The last section deals with motivation and personality-style questions. These need to be answered honestly, reflecting your motivation for your career in pharmacy. (Reproduced with permission.)

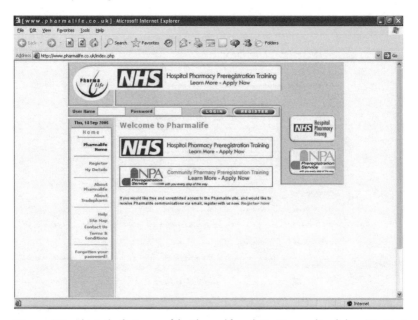

Figure 14 This is the first page of the Pharmalife website. You need to click on 'Register' to register yourself as a user.

Figure 15 On this page, you register your personal details. This allows you to access the website.

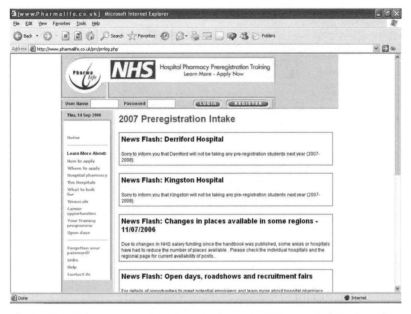

Figure 16   Once you are registered, you then go to the NHS pre-registration front page.

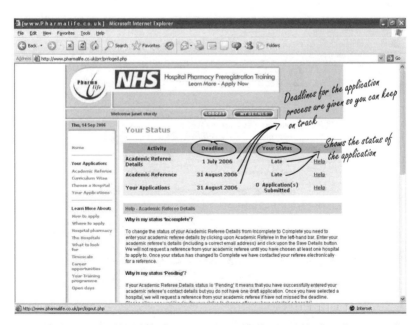

Figure 17   You then log on with your user name and password. This takes you to the application status page.

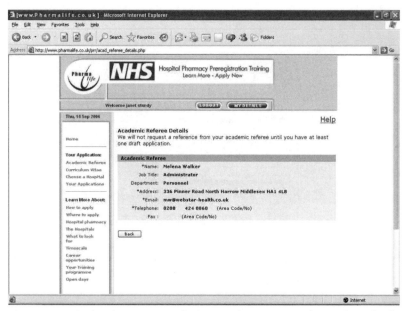

Figure 18 The first thing you are asked to complete is your academic referee details. You must contact your academic referee before putting his/her name down and ask for permission.

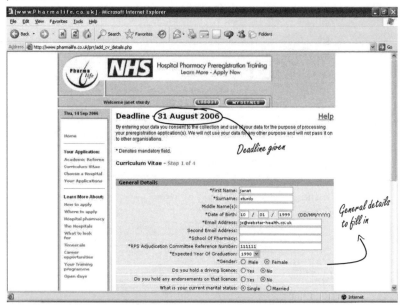

Figure 19 Step 1 of filling out the CV. You then have to fill out a CV. The deadline for this is given. It is very important that you adhere to deadlines. Applying for a job is not like submitting course work – you won't get an extension!

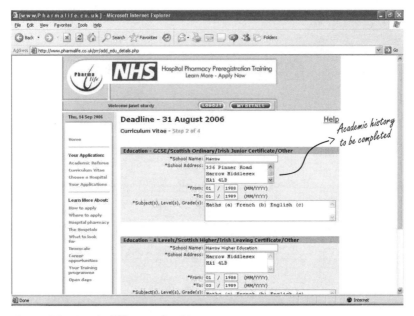

Figure 20 Step 2 of filling out the CV.

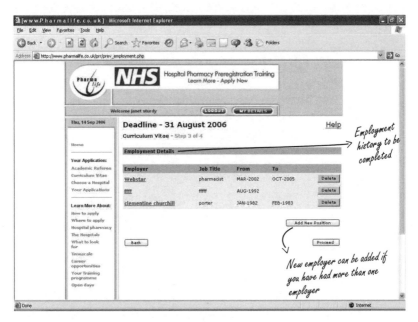

Figure 21 Step 3 of filling out the CV.

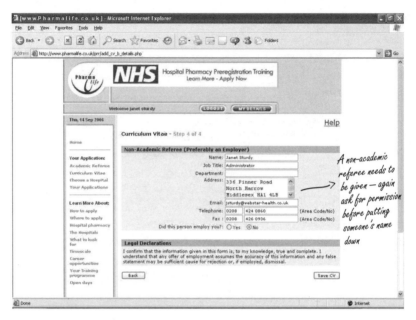

Figure 22   Step 4 of filling out the CV.

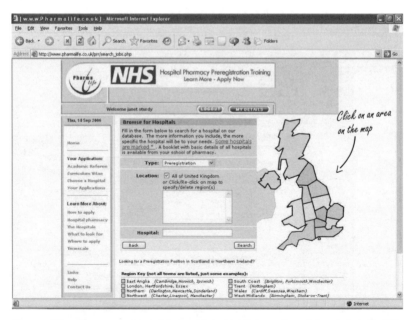

Figure 23   Choose a hospital: this page helps you browse through hospitals in the UK.

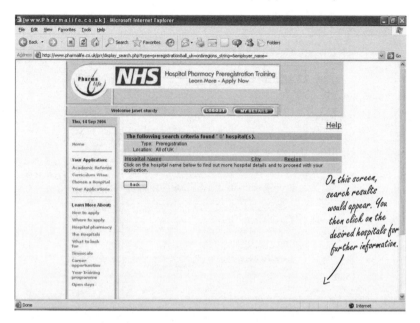

Figure 24 Search results.

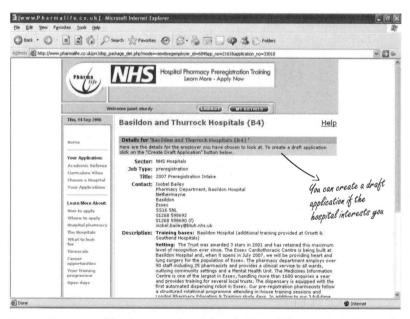

Figure 25 Hospital details: you can then click on the hospital of interest for further details.

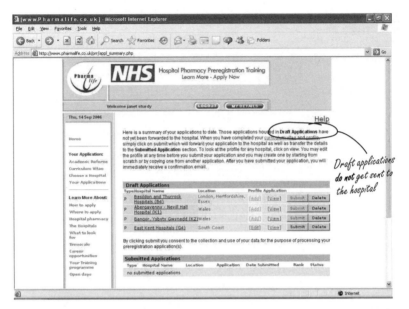

Figure 26 This page shows draft and submitted applications. You can choose to apply to four hospitals in the UK. You can also choose whether you wish to rank your choice. It is advised that you do not rank, or you may be vulnerable to being asked why you chose a particular hospital as your third or fourth choice.

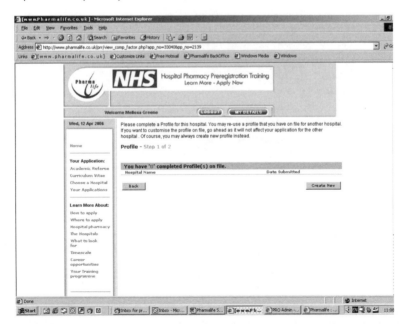

Figure 27 Profile: step 1 of 2. You need to submit a profile for each hospital you are applying to.

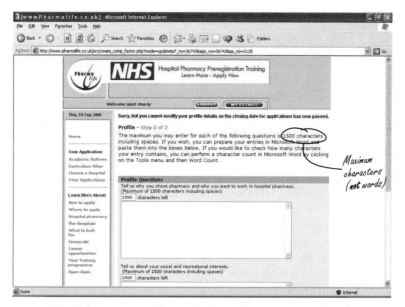

Figure 28 Profile: step 2 of 2. These profile questions need to be carefully thought through before you write and submit this section.

Figure 29 Before you submit your application, a pop-up will appear, asking you to rank the hospital. Avoid doing this, as the hospitals are informed of the ranking and may question you on your choice. Once you submit your application the process is complete. You then need to log on regularly to monitor the progress of your application.

Once stage 2 of the application process is successful, you are then short-listed for an interview. Most students are very excited at this point as they have made it to stage 3 and have beaten most of the competition. Interviews are very daunting and terrifying and should not be taken lightly. The question bank in this book will prepare you well for the types of questions you may be asked at interviews. It is advised that you practise all questions, regardless of the sector in which you are attending an interview. Questions do overlap, and by practising all questions, you will be better equipped on the day. The chapter How to Conduct Yourself on the Day will give you handy tips for the interview so that you can perform at your peak.

Students often face a dilemma when they have successfully completed stage 3 of the application process. Some students are accepted by their second or third choices but want to wait to hear from their first choice. Employers who are not their first choice may then start putting pressure on students to give a verbal commitment on whether they accept the post or not. The Royal Pharmaceutical Society of Great Britain (RPSGB) has released guidelines for students on this (Appendix 1). The RPSGB set a date in October before which students do not have to commit themselves to a pre-registration post. However, it must be noted that this is merely a guideline from the RPSGB: employers may not wish to adhere to this and may continue to put pressure on students to give a prompt reply. I would advise that students weigh their options carefully in this instance. In the past students have declined offers from renowned companies waiting for hospital replies but in the end have been rejected from the hospital of their choice. This leaves students in a poor position and they then have to go through the clearing process.

If you are ever in doubt, and unsure about your rights regarding accepting posts, it is best to speak to a representative of the RPSGB and follow that advice.

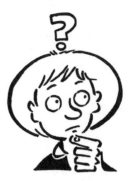

What are employers looking for?

The million-dollar question for any student applying for a pre-registration position is: what are employers looking for?

For this chapter, it was thought that it would be most informative if prospective employers were asked this question.

The pre-registration recruiters from two large community pharmacy companies, two well-known teaching hospitals and an industrial company, which is very popular with students, were asked this question.

WHAT DOES YOUR COMPANY/HOSPITAL LOOK FOR IN A PRE-REGISTRATION STUDENT?

Community pharmacy 1

'We look for drive in our students. What makes them want to work in our sector? Enthusiasm is important for us. If the students do not show any interest in us, we are not interested in them! Communication skills and organisational skills are also of value to us. We look for basic clinical knowledge. For example, if you were to sell ibuprofen over the counter, what would you look out for?

'We want our students to be aware of issues around running a business. They should have a commercial awareness, for example, how to increase sales, how to plan staff so that there is maximum benefit, how to cope with losses and any strategies that should be used to increase profit.'

Community pharmacy 2

'We are looking for students this year that already closely match our company values. We are looking for people who we can develop in the future. Our values define the kind of company we want to be, the way we treat each other and get things done and what our motivations and standards are. These are the qualities that mirror our company values: passionate, challenging and brave, listening and respectful, acting decisively, accountable and celebrating success.'

Hospital 1

'We are looking for students who can fit in well in a team and our workplace. They need to fit in well with other pre-regs. We are looking for a personality and we want them to be flexible in their approach. We want them to be sociable, stand out, be a quick learner and we are also looking for academically sound students.'

Hospital 2

'We are looking for highly enthusiastic individuals who work well in a team and can fit in well in our pharmacy department. Having experience in a hospital setting is definitely a plus point and it displays favour towards hospital pharmacy. We really want students with a personality and who are passionate about their career and wish to progress well in the future. We want students with career aspirations and who are willing to excel. We look for many transferable skills such as teamwork, time management and organisational skills.'

Industry

'We look for academically strong individuals who have a range of competencies and transferable skills. We would favour students who have some research experience and we would be very encouraged to see students who have done a previous summer placement in the industrial sector.'

CAN YOU GIVE ANY ADVICE ON THE APPLICATION FORMS?

Community pharmacy 1

'Our application form is online. Spelling and grammar are something we really look out for. On one of the application forms, a student had misspelt "shift work" by omitting the letter "f"! One piece of advice is that if students plan their answer on a word processor, they can run a grammar and spell-check on it before they copy it on the actual form online. We may penalise for poor spelling and grammar. Do put down all your work experience, even if it is voluntary. This then shows us that you have experience in areas others than pharmacy, which is a plus point. If you are going to be doing a third-year placement before you submit your application form, please do include this in your work experience and mention that you will be doing this the following summer. This gives us an insight of your experience by the time you start your pre-registration.'

Community pharmacy 2

'The application form is a save-and-return form and any student who does not know the answer straight away should go away and research before completing it.'

Hospital 1

'Please avoid mobile text language such as "u 2" or "r u frm lndn". If you have poor grammar, write the answers out in a Word document and then paste it into your application form. To make your application form stand out, it would be very useful to us if students pointed out what they can give to us! If students have put their time and effort into writing their forms, it really does show. One thing to point out to students is that we know what student language sounds like. So if you are copying and pasting from a website, we can catch you out. We want you to be yourself and use your own language style; otherwise it makes no sense to us! When we see applicants and we hear their English, we often say to ourselves: "Did this student really write his/her own application form?" So my advice is: be true to yourself. There should be some kind of match between application form language and the language used at the interviews.'

Hospital 2

'On the application forms we are looking for good English, spelling and grammar. Having previous experience at the hospital will be of great benefit to the student. Be original; explain why you are studying pharmacy. So many students will say the same thing when it comes to why they chose pharmacy – we really want to hear something novel and different! Use your common sense.

'We like students with a wide experience as it shows commitment, so tell us about your non-pharmacy experience as well! I know it may be hard for you to understand this but we can detect lies! Be yourself and do not give us false information. One year a student said she loved to do yoga in her spare time. Bad luck for her that one of the interviewers was a pro at yoga. So the interviewer asked the student: "Can you show me the lotus position?" This threw the student as she had no idea – not to mention how embarrassed she was that she had lied. By telling just one little lie, she sabotaged getting a place. So it really is not worth it!

'Academically we do not look down on you if you do not have predictions of getting a first or a 2:1. We look more for practical ability and experience. A good application form gets an interview!'

Industry

'We do not have application forms for our company. We ask students to submit their CVs. My first point is: please don't tell me about the company I work for! I already know everything about it. Tell us about yourself: what you are like as a person, what you do in your spare time, what types of skill you have, what you can offer our company, why we should employ you. Really sell yourself and try and display enthusiasm about why you want to be an industrial pharmacist.'

CAN YOU GIVE ANY INTERVIEW ADVICE? ANY DOS AND DON'TS?

Community pharmacy 1

'We are starting a novel approach for recruiting in pharmacy which involves team-building games. This comprises a discussion group where we monitor each student's interaction with colleagues. This would then be followed by a mini-interview and the day would be finished off with a group activity.

'We are looking for a cross of the following skills: teamwork, confidence, approach to difficult situations, reactions to various situations, communication, interaction and, most importantly, drive. So, bearing all this in mind, we try to get a cross of these skills and see if the individual can fit in with our company.

'Regarding the mini-interview, we would strongly suggest that students keep a copy of their application form. One piece of advice I would like to give all students is: please tell the truth – you will get found out! Even though the interview is formal, we like our students to feel at ease and really want to see their personality come through. Yes or no answers really won't do; we really want to see the personality! If you do not know about the company you are applying for, it does reflect badly on you – use the internet, go on the company's website.

'The group activity is competency-based. We are looking for individuals who can work well in a team but who are also capable of working on their own. We want to see how individuals control certain situations; that's where their true personality comes out. We use non-pharmacy examples in these exercises as it allows students to think outside the box. We are looking for students who stand out.'

Community pharmacy 2

'With regard to the interviews, students are reminded to follow instructions on what is required of them at interview (i.e. preparing a 10-minute presentation: some attend and say they have forgotten it). Other areas that need to be better are:

- Attending on time
- Telephoning to cancel if not attending
- Telephoning if they are going to be late.'

Hospital 1

'Very standard, but important advice: first, be yourself. Try not to be nervous, especially if you say that you can handle stressful situations well! It is a short interview, once you are inside! Do not pretend you know or have done something because you soon get found out. Try not to "blag". Come early and make the effort to find out where you are going. Contact us if you are going to be late, and this will show you in a positive light as it demonstrates that you are responsible. Try and understand what you have read. Do not just mention buzzwords such as '*Agenda for Change*' and not know about it! Finally there is not really much point talking about community issues such as MURs in hospital.'

Hospital 2

'Look at how you conduct yourself. All eyes are on you and it is very important that you conduct yourself well and that you come across as confident. How you cope with question-answering is very important. This demonstrates many skills which we will be marking you on. We want you to show common sense when answering questions: even if you do not know the answer, use your common sense and tell us how you would go about answering if you had the correct resources.

'We don't expect you to know everything – we know you have limitations, but sometimes students do not know their limitations and push themselves to answer these questions incorrectly. If you don't know, then be honest both to yourself and to us.

'Communication skills are a skill which usually comes out in an interview. Students who are confident, talk clearly and concisely and give correct information usually stand out above others.

'We expect students to participate in continuing professional development (CPD), thus students should be aware how this works, what it is and have views on it – explain CPD and answer individually with examples.

'We want you to draw attention to your attributes. What can you offer our pharmacy department? This is something students should think of when they are preparing for their interviews.

'When talking about your work experience, bring in evidence: what have you learnt from work experience? Give us examples of this and maybe some points of reflection too.'

Industry

'Expect technical questions as well the typical general questions. The typical questions are usually on pharmaceutics, so do revise your pharmaceutics notes! We ask about solid dosage forms and solubility, but there is a whole range of areas which students would be expected to answer, as they would have covered it during their undergraduate degree.'

HOW DO YOU SELECT YOUR STUDENTS FOR INTERVIEW AND THEN FOR A PRE-REG PLACE?

Community pharmacy 1

'Students are selected on their application forms and their references. Based on how students score on the day and whether they stand out and meet our company's requirements, we offer a pre-reg place.'

Community pharmacy 2

'Students are selected initially on their application score for interview and then their interview score for a pre-reg place. We have a pre-agreed cut-off point: those who score below this point will receive a decline letter and those with the highest scores will be offered a position first.'

Hospital 1

'We pick different players on our team, like a football team. We can't have two goalkeepers. What we try and do is pick different personality types as we are aware of the dynamics at the workplace. To avoid conflicts we look for a mixture, e.g. leaders, followers, people who keep things together, and this makes up our successful pre-reg team.'

Hospital 2

'Students are selected for an interview according to their application form and references. Once they come for an interview, we look for commitment, personality and a teamplayer.'

Industry

'We are looking for students with personality and we are very keen to take on team-players. We like students who are grateful and enthusiastic. Listen to the question and think! Do not reel off answers which you have learnt off by heart! Try and think and answer the question according to the situation. We want students who have a professional approach. On the day do find out where you are going: it seems highly unprofessional otherwise. The interview is based on a point-scoring system to see how closely the students matches the job description, so be sure you are familiar with that document when you are preparing for your interview.'

CAN YOU GIVE ANY GENERAL ADVICE TO STUDENTS?

Community pharmacy 1

'Be yourself! If you are not, we do soon find out. Be comfortable and feel at ease. Talk, but do not talk nonsense or unnecessarily. If you do not know the answer to a question, say honestly "I don't know" or " I know where to find the answer". Do not make up rubbish! One year we had a student and we asked him what were the contraindications of ibuprofen. He honestly told us that he could not answer the question. The same evening, I received an e-mail from the same student with the answer to the question. We hired him. The fact that he followed up after the interview displayed his conscientiousness and enthusiasm for his career.'

Hospital 1

'Students often become stressed about the clinical questions at a hospital interview. We do not ask our students clinical questions as we train them, bearing in mind that they have a zero baseline when it comes to clinical knowledge, so we build all our pre-reg students up together. We want our students to have an insight into real issues and have opinions on them. We expect students to read the *Pharmaceutical Journal* and they should be aware of the latest advances in pharmacy.'

Hospital 2

'Ensure you do adequate background reading. That really is the best way to prepare; read all the relevant information on advances in the world of pharmacy. The *Pharmaceutical Journal* is a great read and it can keep you abreast of the latest issues.

'We want students to appreciate the ethos of the workplace.

'Try not to be overly humorous at the interview. It really does not impress us!

'Try not to show that you rank our hospital as your second or third choice. We might give preference to students who have put us down as their first choice.'

Industry

'If students have been on our open day, we do remember them and it displays commitment. We like our students to be professional and respectful towards others. On the day of the interview, we watch our students over lunch to see how they interact with each other. This often gives us an insight into the student's personality.'

SUMMARY

From reading what prospective employers are looking for, you can hopefully see a pattern. They all want to employ an individual who displays confidence, has excellent social skills and would fit in well in their team. Although this may sound straightforward, it may be hard to display these qualities in an interview setting. The best advice is to be yourself. Take a moment to think about the answer to a question before answering it and try to make good eye contact and project your voice well.

Your application form or CV is the gateway to getting an interview, so you must allocate enough time when you are completing it. Write your answers in a Word document and run a spell and grammar check so that you have one less thing to worry about.

On the day you must try to sell yourself. Those 30–40 minutes are your moment of glory. You really have to iterate your transferable skills and give good honest examples of how you feel you have attained those skills. All employers are looking for an excellent team-worker, a good communicator, someone who can multitask, someone who can work well alone and under pressure, as well as having good time management and organisational skills. One piece of advice is to list all the transferable skills on a piece of paper and then think of scenarios you have come across which would display those skills. When thinking of examples, try to include non-pharmacy-related examples as well as pharmacy-related examples. This gives some variety and shows the interviewers that you have a range of experiences. Using non-pharmacy examples also lets your personality shine through. So the key is really to have a mixture of both pharmacy and non-pharmacy examples in your interviews.

Lastly, as many employers have said, be honest. Lies can be detected and they really can show you up and hinder your chances of getting the place you really wanted.

Hopefully this chapter has given you some useful tips on the application form and the interview process – so get cracking and do your homework!

How to conduct yourself on the day

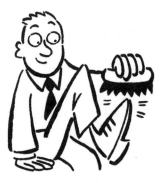

The day for which you have been preparing finally dawns. It would be a good idea to get a good night's sleep the night before the interview so that you are fresh to take on the challenge of the interview.

Employers are well aware that the interview process may be daunting for students, as for some this may be the first time they have been interviewed. Employers are also sensitive of the stress and the implications for a student of being unsuccessful at an interview. Try and calm yourself as this will demonstrate to the interview panel that you are in control and also demonstrates the skill of being able to cope in stressful situations.

A good way to calm down is by preparing your clothes the night before and visualising how you will impress the panel the next day. Think to yourself that you are the best person for the job and that your employers need you, not the other way round. If you begin to think about how badly you want the job or that you will be nervous answering questions asked by three panel members, this will just make you more nervous and may hinder your performance on the day.

PREPARATION BEFORE THE INTERVIEW

Know yourself

Of course you have a copy of your application form or your covering letter! This is the time to re-read what you wrote. Try to think about it from the employer's point of view. What are your strong and your weak points? What areas might need clarification? Is there anything not on the form that you think they need to know?

Everything you put in your application is fair game for an interview question, so be prepared to expand on any of the information you have given.

Know the job

Re-read the job description. Talk to people doing the same type of job. List the skills and qualities needed and think about the evidence you can draw from your experience to demonstrate that you have these skills.

The more you can demonstrate that you know about the job, the more likely it is that the employer will believe you when you say you are well suited to it.

Know the organisation

Find out as much as you can about the employer. Visit the organisation's website or try the employer information files in the Careers Service. Try and get hold of the annual report. Companies often have mission/vision statements or key principles: try to think of situations in your own life which demonstrate those principles.

Keep your eyes on the news for any stories about the organisation or its sector. Make a note of the facts and try to form opinions.

Many organisations hold presentations. As well as being a useful source of information, these events can be an opportunity to get some inside knowledge about the organisation and meet some of the people with whom you may be working if you are successful.

Know the details

Check the time of the interview, the date, the location (it may not be at the employer's offices) and the name and job title of the interviewer. It is probably best to take the letter inviting you to the interview along with you. Have the phone number available in case anything goes wrong.

Make sure you know how to get there and how long it will take. Make sure that you have the right clothes washed and ironed and that you have set your alarm clock. Try to get a good night's sleep.

ON THE DAY

One of the most important things is to ensure that you look presentable: first impressions count. Although it may seem obvious, make sure your hair is tidy, your fingernails are clean and your shoes are polished. For male candidates, a suit is strongly recommended. For female candidates a suit or smart dress is highly advisable.

Although some of you may strongly wish to wear them, trainers are not at all professional shoe wear. Please do try and invest in smart, professional shoes.

Female candidates should refrain from wearing large dressy earrings at the interview. Smart studs or small hoops are regarded as appropriate and elegant. (This is also true for male candidates.)

If you have more than one piercing, try to be professional in how you present this on the day of the interview.

Make sure you know where your interview is being held. For example, if you are applying in a trust, find out at which hospital the interview is being held. Always allow plenty of time for the journey; public transport may fail you on the one occasion when you need it to be at its most efficient.

Try and avoid speaking to other candidates in the waiting room, unless you want to talk to them about the weather! It may make you feel more nervous as you may have the impression that they are better than you and that they may get the position instead of you! However, do not appear unfriendly – smile at fellow colleagues so that you seem pleasant and sociable.

It is inevitable that you will be feeling nervous. Nevertheless, try and keep your mind occupied with other things before the interview. Last-minute reading of the *Pharmaceutical Journal* or the *British National Formulary* (BNF) will only make you more nervous. It may be better to read the paper instead!

Remember to speak slowly and clearly; sometimes we fail to realise how much we mumble in a stressful situation. It is also a good idea to pause for about 5–10 seconds after the interviewer has asked a question. This shows the interviewer that you think before you answer and it also gives you time to structure your answer in your head.

Never be ashamed to admit your deficiencies. If the interviewer asks you a question which you are unable to answer, it is best to admit that you are having difficulty in answering the question rather than waffling on with no clear direction.

Recently in an interview a student was asked the side-effects of gentamicin. The student was honest and said that he did not know the answer. The interviewers appreciated this and the rest of the interview went smoothly. The student then went home, looked up the side-effects of gentamicin in the BNF and e-mailed the answer to the interviewers. The panel were extremely impressed by the candidate's conscientiousness and the student was offered a pre-registration placement.

SOME DOS AND DON'TS FOR INTERVIEWS

Dos

- Dress to impress – suits are a safe option
- Arrive at least 15 minutes before the interview time – if you are running late, let the interviewer know, as this shows good time management skills
- Switch off your mobile phone
- Shake hands firmly
- Ask before you sit down
- Sit up and don't slouch; try and portray good body language. This tells a lot about a person
- Make eye contact when you are speaking and being spoken to; when you are addressing a panel, concentrate more on the person who has asked the question, but keep on looking at the others to help them be engaged and feel involved
- Be enthusiastic
- Sell yourself – talk about all your transferable skills and give original examples. Give both pharmacy- and non-pharmacy-related examples, as this will help you stand out more
- Use proper, non-colloquial language, as this demonstrates good communication skills
- Be confident; try to project your voice and vary your tones. Use occasional hand gestures, when appropriate
- Ask intellectual questions; always ask a question or two at the end, as this shows your enthusiasm and motivation. However, do not ask about the salary or how many holidays you will get! Try to ask questions related to training or, to be really original, challenge one of the interviewers!
- Close the interview positively; don't rush to leave the room. It looks very unprofessional

Don'ts

- Chewing gum is very unprofessional
- Try not to smoke beforehand as you will smell of smoke!
- Don't be shy and timid. Project your voice and display your confidence
- Try not to appear desperate for the position!
- Do not give unconstructive criticism about former colleagues or lecturers or friends – this will demonstrate that you are not a good team-player

- Lying will not be tolerated by any employer. Answer questions as honestly as you can
- Explain your answers. Do not restrict your answers to simply 'yes' or 'no'

It will be all right on the night, as they say. Smile frequently as this lets your personality shine through. However, do not giggle unnecessarily, as this may annoy the interviewers!

Try to enjoy the process as much as you can. Just be yourself and knock their socks off!

What if it all goes wrong?

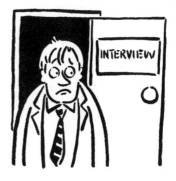

You may feel disheartened if you do not secure a pre-registration placement with the company or hospital you wished to work for. However, thank your lucky stars that you have a placement, even if it is not with your first choice. As stated before, what you learn and experience in your placement is down to you. You may need to be proactive at times and push for new experiences. That is not a bad thing. You may learn more this way. You are still lucky to have acquired a place and you can now get on with it and concentrate on your career.

If you have been unsuccessful in securing any place, try not to panic, although that is easier said than done. It is appreciated that the rest of your life depends on having a placement and not having one slows down the whole process of qualifying as a pharmacist.

If you still have not got a pre-registration place despite going through the clearing process, you can register with the National Pharmaceutical Association (NPA). This represents all community pharmacies except Boots the Chemist and has a web-based pre-registration service where you can register your details (www.npa.co.uk). Your details will be sent to potential employers who will contact you if they're interested. You can also browse vacancy listings.

The other option is to reapply the following year and take a year out. In this year out, you should try and do something constructive, so you can add it to your CV in a positive light.

Currently, there is no time limit set by the Pharmaceutical Society on how many years you have, after graduating with a Masters in Pharmacy degree, before you have to undertake a pre-registration trainee position. Therefore, you can keep on trying! It may seem like an uphill struggle, but if you are really determined to qualify as a pharmacist, you will have to persevere.

Remember, you can contact independent pharmacies as well as all other sectors of pharmacy. The main advice to reiterate here is not to confine yourself to one region – apply all over the UK.

Reading up for the interviews

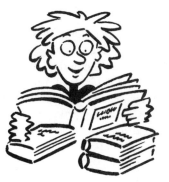

Today's pharmacist plays a large and important role in the delivery of quality health care. Pharmacists are at the frontline in health care and, unless they are working for the industrial or private sector, pharmacists will always be involved with the NHS.

The interviews are a very crude method of assessing whether one is suitable for a particular post. Questions regarding the novel approaches in pharmacy and using your hypothetical professional judgement are inevitable. One can only prepare for this by engaging in analysing the latest topics and problems in pharmacy. Reading around the latest developments in the profession is the obvious and easiest method of doing this.

This chapter will direct you to various documents with which you should be familiar before you attend your pre-registration interviews.

It cannot be overemphasised how important it is for you to be up to date with current issues in pharmacy and be aware of key developments in the NHS. You should also have a fair idea of how the NHS works. If you have not already done a placement in the NHS, try and visit a hospital pharmacy for a day. Theoretically knowing how a hospital works is one thing, but seeing how it functions practically is another.

The *Pharmaceutical Journal* is the most appropriate reference source for pharmacy students and pharmacists to keep abreast of the latest advances in pharmacy. Accessing the *Pharmaceutical Journal* is very simple: log on to www.pjonline.com and search the journal on a weekly basis for current issues. New guidance is always being published, so you need to keep up to date. Prospective employers are very interested in your views on current issues. It is thus very important that you read around subject areas and form opinions and arguments around them, so that you are fully prepared for any questions you may be asked. Another excellent resource for keeping up to date is the internet. If you key in 'current issues in pharmacy' to a well-known search engine, such as Google (ensure you ask for pages from the UK), you will have a extensive reading list to keep you busy!

Apart from the *Pharmaceutical Journal*, there are a few documents that you need to read before your interviews. There are also a few organisations which you need to be aware of and have an idea of the work they are undertaking. It is appreciated that it is a great deal of reading; however, you are not expected to read each document cover to cover. Reading the summaries of each document and maybe homing in on more interesting issues would be of immense benefit. Again, formulating your opinions on each topic would be very advantageous.

Continuing professional development (CPD) is a current hot topic in the pharmacy world. It would be of benefit if you carried out research in this area and prepared some examples on how you would conduct CPD and how you participate in reflection.

There are two informative articles in the *Pharmaceutical Journal* on interview skills and CPD. Check out the links below:

- http://www.pjonline.com/pdf/cpd/pj_20020427_interview.pdf
- http://www.pharmj.com/pdf/features/pj_20020525_mandatorycpd.pdf

Below is a checklist of current issues in pharmacy. This list is not exhaustive, so please do search the Pharmaceutical Journal for further up-to-the-minute issues. The extra reading will be supplementary – you can never read enough!

CURRENT ISSUES IN PHARMACY

- *The NHS Plan* and *Pharmacy in the Future*: you need to understand how these involve pharmacy
- *Spoonful of Sugar* (medicines management): you need to appreciate what medicines management is and how it can influence pharmacy and the NHS
- *Vision for Pharmacy*: this is a follow-on from *Pharmacy in the Future* to further developments in pharmacy implementing *Pharmacy in the Future*
- National Institute for Clinical Excellence (NICE): you need to understand what this organization is. Read a few guidelines produced by NICE (www.nice.org.uk). Try and understand what the organisation does and have a view on the guidelines it has produced
- National Service Frameworks (NSFs): what are these? Again, try and understand what they do (www.doh.gov.uk/nsf/index.htm). How can NSFs help with prescribing?
- Pharmacist's prescribing: various articles in the *Pharmaceutical Journal* explain pharmacist's prescribing
- CPD: there are many articles in the *Pharmaceutical Journal* regarding CPD, as mentioned before.

- Patient group directions (PGDs): search the *Pharmaceutical Journal* to further your understanding on this. How are PGDs different from supplementary prescribing?
- Office of Fair Trading (OFT) report: search this in the *Pharmaceutical Journal* – what is the OFT? Which sector of pharmacy does it affect?
- Improving medication safety: this is hot off the press so make sure you get to grips with this
- Guidance will be published soon on changes in the prescribing of controlled drugs, prompted by the Harold Shipman case. Please keep your eyes peeled for this one!
- Hot topics: *Agenda for Change* is the current hot topic among today's pharmacy team so search on Google and the *Pharmaceutical Journal* and read up on the most current information

You will come across many other terms and phrases when you go through the question bank, and I suggest you look them up on the *Pharmaceutical Journal* website.

Don't panic! It is appreciated that a lot of information is given, but interviewers do not expect you to know the contents of each document in great detail. Employers are not testing your knowledge – they want you to have an awareness of current issues in the NHS. This also demonstrates to them your ability to communicate clearly and express opinions on subject matters. This is tested because, when you are a practising pharmacist, you will be making decisions independently so you must have views, opinions and arguments and be able to back them up with evidence.

Question bank introduction

This is the grand finale of the book – a series of real interview questions asked over the past 4 years in hospital and community interviews. There are a few industry questions; however, not many students had applied to the industrial sector, and therefore the proportion of questions submitted to the bank is less. Nevertheless, the general miscellaneous-type questions will be generic at any interview, so it would be beneficial to practise them for an industrial interview.

Sample answers to some questions within each category are given after the set of questions. This is to give students a guide to the type of answers to be thinking about. They are solely the view of the author: they are by no means advising students on the correct way to answer questions. As mentioned before, they are thought-provoking and aim to stimulate students' own thinking.

Question bank

HOT OFF THE PRESS!

○ Are there any issues in the media that are related to pharmacy?

○ What are the current issues in pharmacy? Do you read any articles?

○ What can you tell us about the recent changes and developments in pharmacy?

○ What are the current problems in pharmacy? How do you think they can be improved?

○ Do you read the *Pharmaceutical Journal* (www.pjonline.com)?

○ Comment on a recent article which you read in the *Pharmaceutical Journal*.

○ What have you recently read in the *Pharmaceutical Journal* regarding community pharmacy?

○ Are there any issues in the media that are related to pharmacy? What are your views on the deregulation of statins from POM to P?

○ How do you keep up to date with current pharmacy issues?

○ What can you tell us about the recent changes and developments in pharmacy?

○ Have you read any interesting articles with regard to new drugs?

○ Is there anything going on in pharmacy or the NHS?

○ Tell us about an article you have read recently.

○ What do you read to keep up to date about pharmacy issues?

○ Name a NICE guideline you have recently read. What do you think about it?

○ Do you think that herbal medicines (complementary therapy) are becoming more important?

○ Do you know of any clinical trials that have been carried out in children? (This is only if you are applying to a specific paediatric hospital)

The key to help answer these questions is to be up to date with the latest pharmacy focuses. The *Pharmaceutical Journal* is one resource which can help you with this. Keep up to date by accessing the journal online – www.pharmj.com.

The better student will also have personal opinions on the issues, rather than merely listing them.

HOT OFF THE PRESS!

Remember to read the Pharmaceutical Journal!

○ Do you read any articles? Name a recent one you have read and tell us about it.

Yes, I regularly read the Pharmaceutical Journal. Recently I read an article about the NHS specification for emergency hormonanal contraception (EHC). The NHS allows for the supply of levonorgestrel EHC in line with the requirements of a local patient group direction. Pharmacies are required to provide a user-friendly, non-judgemental, client-centred and confidential service.

Once you have explained the article, you can then give your views on what you think about this service.

○ What have you recently read in the journal about community pharmacy?

Recently an article was published in the Pharmaceutical Journal regarding the need for an allocated budget for pharmacists in primary care.

'A dedicated budget should be allocated to pharmacy to avoid a wrangle with the medical profession and PCTs [primary care trusts] charged with the responsibility to implement extended medicines management,' according to the Independent Pharmacy Federation. The PCT should commission enhanced services from a 'national menu' and purchase services deemed to be required as a result of a robust local pharmaceutical care needs assessment.

Again, students should give their opinions and views on this matter, or whichever matter they choose to discuss about.

TEAMWORK

○ Can you describe a time when you worked in a team and it was successful?

○ When have you had to build relationships with people you are unfamiliar with? How did you manage to do this? Could you improve on this?

○ Do you work well on your own or are you a team-player?

○ Why is the team-working skill important in a setting such as hospital pharmacy?

○ Do you prefer to be a leader of a team or are you a more passive member?

○ Do you work well on your own? Explain.

○ What position do you see yourself in a team? i.e. a team leader or follower?

○ If someone in a team is dominating the rest of the team, how would you handle this?

○ Explain a situation when you had to work in a team. What went well and what did not?

○ You are working in a group of five people. You have five days left for three joined assignments to be handed in, what do you do?

○ Describe a situation where you have worked within a team, something has gone wrong and you have contributed to solving the problem.

○ Tell me what things are important in a team.

○ Describe when you have worked as part of a team. What was your role? Was it a success?

○ How would you get other members of the team to pull their weight and fulfil their role if they are not working as hard as they are meant to?

The concept of teamwork applies to a group of people, perhaps with varying backgrounds, who have a common goal.

Teamwork is a transferable skill which is paramount in any professional role, especially health care, where you will be part of a multidisciplinary team.

The way to answer these questions is to prepare examples where you have worked together with people, whether personally, academically or in your part-time job.

You may have been part of a charity fund-raising event, you may have had to do a group presentation, or maybe you worked with a variety of people in your part-time job to complete a set task.

Once you have prepared some examples, try and think what went well and what you could have improved on. By relaying this extra information to your interviewer, you will demonstrate that you reflect upon your actions – a good way to earn extra points!

TEAMWORK

Point to note: teamwork is when everyone is working towards a common objective. Let's look at the example of the staff working in a hospital:

- ○ **Doctors,** who are involved in making major clinical decisions on patients

- ○ **Pharmacists,** who can give advice to doctors on the correct medicine management of the patient

- ○ **Nurses,** who provide more pastoral and one-to-one care of the patient

- ○ **Physiotherapists,** who aim to improve a patient's mobility after a long stay in hospital

- ○ **Auxiliaries,** who give patients their meals

- ○ **Cleaners,** who maintain the sanitation of the hospital so all the team can carry out their duties

The list goes on! All these people have different roles; however, they all have one common objective – to help make the patient better!

- ○ Why would others want you on their team?

Everyone in a team is working towards the same purpose. When working with a group of people, it is important that you express your views effectively on how to achieve the objective. In contrast to this, one also needs to be able to listen to what others in the team have to say. I would therefore sell myself by saying that I can communicate my opinions confidently, whilst having the ability to listen to others, and take their advice on board.

○ Can you tell me a situation where you had to work in a group with a difficult person? How did you handle the situation? What did you learn from this? (Some of you may have encountered such a situation in a Saturday job. Others may have had a particularly difficult member of a sports team. If you have never been in such a scenario, then you must have been in a group of friends where someone was difficult! Remember, if you are in an unfamiliar situation, try to apply familiar concepts to it.)

In my previous vacation employment, I was in charge of a group of security personnel in a stadium. Every individual was given a time during the day when they could take their breaks, which had to be strictly adhered to. One particular member did not adhere to this, and his actions were letting down other members of the team. I took this member of staff to a private area and explained to him in a calm but firm manner why it was important to stick to the timings he was given, after which the matter was resolved. This taught me how to deal with different members of a team. It would have been easy for me to humiliate him in front of his colleagues. However, by rationally talking to him in a private setting, I maintained his honour as a valuable team member.

○ What does 'being a good team-player' mean to you?

In my opinion, being a good team-player means doing your best to try to achieve the common goal which all team members share. If I am the team leader, I would make the decisions which I feel to be in the team's best interest, after taking into consideration the views of all team members. If I am not the team leader, I would make my opinions known to the other members, whilst also respecting their views. I think the most important ingredient of being a good team-player is to have the ability to work with others, who will probably have different personalities and backgrounds to me.

○ If someone in your team is being dominating, how would you handle the situation? (This is a difficult question! If you are not the team leader, you could consider speaking to others about the matter. However, if they do not feel the same as you, then **you** may be letting the team down by starting unnecessary rifts! Therefore, you must be careful in your approach to this type of question.)

If I felt like this, then I would approach the team leader about my concerns in a confidential setting. The team leader should be a trustworthy person, who is able to keep such things in confidence. I would suggest that there should be a more even delegation of tasks, so that everyone feels involved in the team, thus improving team morale. Furthermore, it may be a good idea to do some simple team-building exercises, such as a social night out, which can help to resolve any tension that could be building up within the team.

ACADEMIA

○ Why did you choose to study pharmacy?

○ What are your favourite subjects at university and why?

○ What are the worst and most enjoyable things about your degree course?

○ What have you found easy and what have you found difficult in your degree?

○ What have you found difficult at university and how have you organised yourself to tackle the problem?

○ What have you enjoyed most about your MPharm programme so far?

○ What would you change in your degree?

○ If you could improve your pharmacy course, what would you do?

○ How would you make changes to the pharmacy practice element of your course?

○ What did you do in your final-year project? What went well? What didn't go so well? What did you learn from this?

○ What did you cover during your third year? What did you enjoy and what not?

○ Why did you choose to do a research project in this particular subject area?

○ Tell me about your project. How was it a challenge for you and has it developed you in any way?

○ Your research project sounds very demanding. How did you overcome the difficult aspects of it?

○ What project have you recently done? Tell us about the good and bad points of doing a project.

○ Are you interested in research? If so, in what area and why?

○ How has your degree geared you for the pre-reg training year?

○ What are the problems in pharmacy as a profession?

Questions on your degree are usually asked first as they are good icebreakers. It helps you to relax and calm down before they fire the technical questions at you!

Have some pointers in your head so you can easily reel out the information on the day. For example:

Pharmacology interests me as it aids my understanding of how drugs work and how I can predict side-effects. This would help me in a clinical setting in optimising patient care.

Pharmacy is at the forefront of health care and I have wanted to be part of this team since I was at school. To further my interest, I took up various work experience placements, which confirmed my passion for pharmacy.

ACADEMIA

○ Why did you choose to study pharmacy?

Being from a family where health care is paramount, I consciously opted for a career in pharmacy. Chemistry was my forte at school and I wished to pursue a career where I could further my interest in the subject but simultaneously have a profession where I would be involved with patient care. After much research I came to know that pharmacy was the only career where chemistry was a core discipline. To confirm my choice, I decided to undertake some voluntary work at my local pharmacy. I thoroughly enjoyed this experience and this sealed the deal for me!

○ What subjects do you dislike and why? How did you motivate yourself to do well in those subjects?

I find pharmaceutics quite hard; maybe that is why I dislike the subject. I understand the importance of the subject for the pharmacist, therefore I had to try and overcome my fear of the subject. I decided to arrange a meeting with the subject tutor to discuss my issues. My tutor was ever so helpful and gave me study tips for pharmaceutics and recommended some easy-to-read materials. Knowing that pharmaceutics was a pharmacy-specific subject area and one of great significance, these factors motivated me to overcome my dislike of it.

○   What have you found difficult in your degree?

To date I haven't found anything difficult in my degree. I have found various subjects and some pieces of assignments challenging, which is a good thing for me as it keeps me on my toes. I feel difficulty is a perception. We should try not to think of things we cannot do as difficult. We should try and find ways of teasing out problems to make them less complicated.

○   How do you think university life will differ from your pre-registration year?

I feel it will be a great transition from university life to pre-reg, There will be a lot of responsibility attached to the job, the relaxed student life will not be there any more; however there will be some similarities. Although I will have completed my undergraduate degree, I will still be learning, training and reflecting on my learning; in effect I will still be a student.

MOTIVATION

○   How do you motivate yourself?

○   How would you motivate yourself when you are in a rotation that you do not enjoy at all?

○   How do you motivate yourself and your supervisor, if you are both given the same task to do?

○   How would you motivate a team?

○   How would you motivate your staff?

○   Motivating others is a great quality: do you possess it? Give an example.

○   Give an example of a time when you have inspired somebody.

○   You are going into your final year now. What would you do if one of your best friends came up to you and said he/she was fed up of the course and was going to drop out?

○   You are working as a pre-registration pharmacist. What would you do if one of your colleagues came up to you and said he/she was fed up with the job and wanted to quit?

○   Where do you see yourself in 5 years' time?

○   Where do you see yourself in 3 years?

○ What do you think a pharmacist's role is heading towards?

○ What do you think the future holds for pharmacy?

○ Have you thought of any particular area in pharmacy (e.g. cardiac) you would like to specialise in and why?

○ If you were in another time at another place, what do you see yourself doing?

At face value, such questions may seem to be very difficult to answer.

You will only be able to motivate yourself if you have a goal established in your mind. Hence, it is very important that you ask yourself: 'How will this potential job help me achieve my eventual goal?' before you go for interview. Some people's goal will be to become a well-renowned consultant pharmacist; others may have a much more personal goal.

The principles of motivating a team are exactly the same as motivating yourself. Sit the team down, perhaps in a team meeting, and try and establish what the collective goal of the team is. In order to achieve this goal, tasks are divided equally amongst members of the team. It is important to remind members of the team constantly what the eventual goal is.

In essence, if you are asked anything about motivation, you need to start discussing goals!

MOTIVATION

Remember to refer to your goals.

○ How would you motivate yourself?

In my opinion, the key to motivating yourself is to have goals which you want to achieve, whether in your career or life. For me personally, my goal is to become a consultant pharmacist. It is human nature for one's motivation to go through highs and lows. Everyone can suffer from a loss of motivation from time to time, and it is important to recognise and deal with this by constantly reassessing your goals. It may be that you have to change your approach to achieving that goal.

○ You are going into your final year now. What would you do if one of your best friends came up to you and said he/she was fed up of the course and was going to drop out?

In this situation, the first thing I would do is to ask my friend why he/she feels like this and gear my advice accordingly. For example, a female colleague could be having personal issues which are affecting her emotionally, thus leading her to feel this way. Dealing with these problems could help ameliorate her feelings towards the course. A more common situation, however, may be that my colleague has lost her drive for pharmacy. In this instance, I would try to take my colleague back to the time when she was applying for pharmacy to remind her why she wanted to do this course and focus on the rewards a pharmacist gains. These rewards are only a year away!

ETHICS

○ Would you give emergency hormonal contraception (EHC or morning-after pill) to a 14-year-old girl? (There are no clinics or hospital in the area for her to obtain one: you are her only hope.)

○ Name three situations where you would **not** sell EHC. Where would you direct these patients?

○ A 17-year-old girl comes to you asking for Levonelle. What would you like to do before you dispense this drug?

○ You are a pharmacist on duty and you are presented with a prescription in which the dose of the drug is over the range. What would you do? Are you going to dispense this drug or not?

○ A locum comes in smelling of alcohol: what would you do? Are you going to let him/her work or not? Are you going to report him/her to the RPSGB?

○ A man comes to you asking to get a prescription dispensed. He says that he will come to pick it up on the following day. The next day, the patient's aunt comes to collect the prescription. Would you give her the medication?

○ A patient is on a surgical ward complaining of severe right-sided abdominal pain. He is lying absolutely still, in an attempt to minimise the sensation of pain. The doctor thinks the patient is suffering from peritonitis, and wants to prescribe morphine for pain relief. You, being a conscientious pharmacist, remember seeing this patient a week ago complaining of the exact same thing. After seeing various needle scars on his forearms, you suspect that the patient is a heroin addict, and has come into hospital to obtain morphine. How would you handle this situation?

○ With the re-emergence of diseases such as tuberculosis, should we curb the number of people seeking asylum in the UK?

○ A patient who is on holiday from Asia attends Accident & Emergency with profuse haematemesis. Bearing in mind that this patient is not a British citizen, should treatment be given on the NHS?

○ A patient has come to your ward presenting with a chest infection. You develop a good relationship with her, to the point that eventually she says that she feels that she can trust you with anything. The patient goes on to tell you that she has recently been diagnosed with HIV, but she doesn't want you to tell any of the doctors. How would you handle this situation?

○ Do you think people who are overweight/smoke/drink deserve treatment at taxpayers' expense?

○ You are a junior pharmacist in a community pharmacy. You see one of your colleagues (who is also a junior pharmacist) becoming extremely friendly with a woman who initially came in to get a prescription dispensed. They exchange phone numbers and arrange to meet in a bar later that evening. How would you advise this colleague?

○ Do you think we should follow our colleagues in the Netherlands and legalise euthanasia?

ETHICS

We are living in a time when ethical issues are more relevant in medical practice than ever before. Many factors have contributed to this, such as technological advances in the medical field, as well as increased patient education on medical matters. Thus employers are keen to test candidates' ethical judgement.

When confronted by an ethical scenario, the first thing to remember is that any decision you make will have to involve the entire team. Therefore, if you are in a hospital setting, you should consult the other doctors and nurses involved in the patient's care. If in the community setting, speak to the other pharmacists/dispensers/ pharmacy managers.

There is no right answer for an ethical question. As mentioned before, if you are not sure, present each side of the argument and try to be diplomatic.

○ A patient is on a surgical ward complaining of severe right-sided abdominal pain. He is lying absolutely still, in an attempt to minimise the sensation of pain. The doctor thinks the patient is suffering from peritonitis, and wants to prescribe morphine for pain relief. You, being a conscientious pharmacist, remember seeing this patient a week ago complaining of the exact same thing. After seeing various needle scars on his forearms, you suspect that the patient is a heroin addict, and has come into hospital to obtain morphine. How would you handle this situation?

The first thing I would do is inform one of my seniors, perhaps the senior pharmacist, or the consultant doctor. It may be necessary to have a private meeting, which involves the whole team in charge of the patient's care.

With this particular scenario, we first need to confirm whether the patient's symptomatology is consistent with organic illness. This is where the clinical judgement of somebody like a consultant would be useful. If the team unanimously agrees that this patient is not suffering from an organic illness, than the best thing to do is first to discuss this with the patient in a sensitive manner, and try to help him accordingly, perhaps referring to social services, or maybe even psychiatric help, if necessary.

○ You are a junior pharmacist in a community pharmacy. You see one of your colleagues (who is also a junior pharmacist) becoming extremely friendly with a woman who initially came in to get a prescription dispensed. They exchange phone numbers and arrange to meet in a bar later that evening. How would you advise this colleague?

I would wait for a quiet moment to discuss this matter with my colleague. I would have to advise him of his professional responsibility, and tell him that such conduct would make him answerable to higher authorities which could put his career at risk. Weighing up what is on offer, is it really worth putting one's entire career at stake for a potential fling?

CLINICAL

○ You may be asked to identify a drug and its uses and side-effects from a drug chart.

○ Name a clinical disease, how it is managed with drug therapy, what you would monitor and how.

○ What is your favourite drug? How does it work? What are its main side-effects?

○ What are opioid analgesics? Give me the side-effects of an opioid and any counselling you would give your patient.

○ If your patient has been prescribed prednisolone for the first time, how would you counsel your patient?

○ Name an antibiotic. What is it used for? Can you tell us what dose is usually prescribed? What are its main side-effects?

○ What counselling points would you give to a patient on antibiotics?

○ What factors should be considered when prescribing antibiotics to children?

○ What is gentamicin? How would you monitor this drug? Why?

○ Name two NSAIDs: what side-effects do they have?

○ What advice would you give to someone taking an NSAID? What are the side-effects?

○ What are the side-effects of ibuprofen?

○ What is warfarin? Name a few important drugs that warfarin interacts with.

○ Do you know of any other anticoagulants aside from warfarin?

○ Look at this prescription and tell us about it: aspirin 75mg OD, ramipril, GTN spray 1–2 sprays prn, simvastatin 40mg OD. How would you distinguish angina?

○ A patient comes in who has recently been diagnosed with coronary heart disease. The doctor prescribed some drugs. What do you think you need to do? And what advice would you give to the patient?

○ Which drug do you give a patient after a heart attack?

○ What medications would you see on a prescription for a patient diagnosed with heart failure?

○ Look at this prescription and talk us through it: aspirin, atenolol, simvastatin and GTN spray, ramipril. Are the doses correct?

○ What is digoxin indicated for? What do you have to measure with this drug?

○ How does digoxin work?

○ What time of day is best to take enalapril, especially the first dose? What are the main side-effects?

○ What is the usual range of INR? What INR would you expect a patient to have if he/she was taking warfarin for DVT prophylaxis?

○ What are the main classes of drugs used for hypertension? How would you monitor a patient on these drugs?

○ Name three classes of drug used for the treatment of hypertension and give an example of a drug in each class.

○ What is TDM and what is it used for? Can you give some examples of drugs that are monitored in this way?

○ What other drugs, apart from antidiabetics, would you expect to see a diabetic patient taking?

○ Can you name some drugs used in diabetes? Can you name a few of their side-effects?

○ What is the difference between salbutamol and beclometasone inhalers?

○ How would you counsel a patient taking beclometasone inhaler for the first time?

○ What is paroxetine? When would you advise a patient to take it? What counselling would you give the patient on how to take the medicine? The same patient wants to buy St John's wort. Do you sell it?

○ Give an example of an opioid analgesic. What are the different preparations of the drug?

○ What are the dose ranges and different frequencies of dosing for tablets and solutions of this drug?

○ What is temazepam? What legal issues would you expect on the prescription?

○ How would you counsel someone on metronidazole?

○ You are selling Levonelle to a patient. How would you counsel the patient?

○ Does the EHC definitely work?

○ What factors do you need to consider when giving medication to a child as opposed to an adult?

○ In paediatric patients, how do you choose the dose?

○ If a prescription read: flucloxacillin 1 capsule tds for a child, what would you check?

○ What are the issues to consider with medicines and prescribing for the elderly?

○ What would you recommend for glaucoma?

○ Situation: you are on a general medical ward and have to counsel a patient who is elderly and has impaired vision as she is going to be discharged with 6–7 medications. How would you do this?

○ A patient asks for pain relief for toothache. What would you sell and how would you counsel the patient?

○ How would you counsel a patient who has been prescribed eye drops for the first time?

○ How would you make sure eye drops are sterile?

○ A mother comes into your pharmacy and tells you that her 3-year-old daughter's eye is red and stuck together. What do you do?

○ What does cytotoxic mean to you?

○ What is chemotherapy?

○ Why would a cytotoxic drug be prepared in a specialised room?

○ If a woman was given tamoxifen and she asks you what it is for, how would you answer?

○ You mentioned Herceptin as a new drug on the NHS: what is it? How does it work?

○ Referring again to Herceptin, which you know: it's a monoclonal antibody. Do you know how they are made?

○ How would you counsel a patient about taking methotrexate?

○ What would a prescription for a controlled drug look like?

○ What is MST?

○ You said you covered depression in detail at university, can you tell me about its treatments? Apart from SSRIs and SNRIs, have you heard about any new developments? So you have heard of reversible MAO inhibitors? Do you know a few?

○ Why is tuberculosis so prevalent in the area?

○ What other diseases do you think occur commonly in the area?

○ Pharmacokinetics of a tablet: draw a graph, and explain the parameters of a single oral dose and multiple oral doses.

○ Industry: talk about the tableting process. What are the key factors of the drug/powder that you will look at before the process?

○ How would you test the tableting process?

○ What should be the glass transition temperature?

○ Can you tell me what a polymer is and give me an example?

○ If you have a poorly soluble acidic drug, what would you do?

○ Look at this inpatient hospital prescription, identify any problems with the doses and method of administration and check the legality (i.e. name, date, signatures, NHS no.).

○ If a patient is unable to swallow tablets, what could you, as a pharmacist, do to ensure that doses of the drug are not missed?

○ What factors do you need to consider when preparing extemporary preparations?

○ What is the role of the clinical pharmacist?

○ How can pharmacists on wards reduce prescription errors that cause ADRs?

○ What do you look for when reviewing a chart?

○ How do you monitor kidney function?

○ How would you check for renal failure?

○ What are the ideal characteristics of the most commonly seen formulations in the hospital?

○ You walk on to the ward and are given a drug chart for a patient. What do you need to look for?

○ Give two examples of drug interactions.

○ What is TPN? What does it contain?

○ If you have two different drugs to go into a single intravenous line, how do you know if it is safe to put them in together?

○ If a nurse wants to give a number of drugs via intravenous infusion, what factors need to be considered?

○ Would you dispense a prescription with an unusual dose, even though the GP agrees the dose is correct?

○ Can you write out a method of how to make a cup of coffee?

○ Please put these drugs in alphabetical order:

  ● Chloramphenicol
  ● Chlordiazepoxide

- Chlorpromazine
- Chlormethiazine
- Carbamazepine

○ Take a look at the following five prescriptions:

- ranitidine and diclofenac
- amoxicillin and flucloxacillin
- aspirin, atenolol, simvastatin and GTN spray
- metformin and gliclazide
- salbutamol and beclometasone

What classes are they, what are they used for and what would you counsel the patients on?

○ In which reference source may you find stability information of a drug?

These questions can be tough as clinical judgement comes with hands-on experience.

It would be an advantage to have some kind of clinical exposure, whether a Saturday job in a pharmacy, or a vocational placement. If this is not possible for you (and there should be no excuse!) then speak to a pharmacist to discuss relevant clinical issues.

It is important for you to consider what post you are applying for. For example, if you are applying for a job in a psychiatric hospital, it may be beneficial for you to focus on the issues surrounding clozapine. However, bear in mind that patients in such specialist hospitals will also have other systemic illnesses, thus basic pharmacology should not be neglected.

In hospital, students are usually given an inpatient drug chart to comment on. For example, if a patient has a history of a peptic ulcer, and is prescribed ibuprofen for chronic pain, you should be able to comment on the choice of analgesia in this patient.

Medication can be given in a variety of ways: orally, rectally and intravenously. Therefore, it would be wise to know the pros and cons of each route of administration. A popular emerging theme looks at the issue of stability of two or more drugs via an intravenous line. Here your knowledge of basic pharmaceutical science will be of use.

Clinical questions for community pharmacy incorporate scenarios. Listed below are examples of role-plays on common conditions which have been used in previous interviews.

- Head lice
- Cystitis
- Thrush

- Diabetes
- Athlete's foot and diabetes
- Hypertension and cholesterol

Therefore, you will need to brush up on over-the-counter conditions as well as common diseases such as diabetes, hypertension and hyperlipidaemia. You should focus on their diagnosis and treatments.

CLINICAL

Note: Remember to consult your Best New Friend (or BNF!) before the interview. If you are asked about drugs, it will probably be about those that are commonly prescribed, such as medicines for treating hypertension, heart disease and diabetes. It is unlikely you will be asked to give the pharmacokinetics of an obscure drug (unless the interviewers are feeling really mean). They may even ask you to talk about a drug of your choice and this gives you the opportunity to look really smart. However don't let this backfire, as if you choose a drug they'll expect you to know **everything** about it!

◯ A drug chart is shown with the following medications: GTN spray, ramipril, aspirin, atenolol and simvastsin. What do you think is wrong with the patient? Tell me about each drug.

The patient is probably an angina patient. The GTN spray is usually taken when required during an attack and is taken sublingually. A side-effect of GTN can be a throbbing headache.

Ramipril is an ACE-inhibitor and a side-effect of this is a dry cough. If the cough is persistent, the patient can see the GP for an alternative angiotensin II antagonist, such as losartan. This is therapeutically equivalent, but does not have the dry cough as a side-effect.

Atenolol is a beta-blocker and a side-effect of this drug can be vivid dreams. Even though atenolol is water-soluble and does not cross the blood–brain barrier, there is still a chance of it causing this side-effect.

Simvastatin is a lipid-lowering drug. Patients should be counselled to monitor signs of muscle weakness and if they do experience such effects, then they should discontinue the drug. The patient's blood pressure, pulse and cholesterol levels should be taken regularly.

◯ Name an antibiotic. What is it used for? Can you tell us what dose is usually prescribed? What are its main side-effects?

Vancomycin is used for endocarditis and MRSA infections. Doses prescribed depend on renal function and condition; however, normally it is prescribed at 1 g twice daily. Side-effects are nephrotoxicity and ototoxicity.

○ What is your favourite drug? How does it work? What are its main side-effects?

My favourite drug is ibuprofen. It is an NSAID which is believed to work through inhibition of cyclooxygenase (COX), thus inhibiting prostaglandin synthesis. Its analgesic, antipyretic and anti-inflammatory activities are achieved principally through COX-2 inhibition, whereas COX-1 inhibition is responsible for its unwanted effects on platelet aggregation and the gastrointestinal mucosa.

Side-effects include nausea, dyspepsia, gastrointestinal ulceration and bleeding, raised liver enzymes, diarrhoea, headache, dizziness, salt and fluid retention and hypertension.

PROFESSIONAL DEVELOPMENT

○ What is the meaning of CPD? Do you think CPD is beneficial? Why?

○ What is CPD and how will it affect you as a pre-registration student?

○ How do you see clinical governance and CPD to be important in your pre-registration year?

○ What is CPD and what is CE (continuing education)?

○ What is CPD, when have you carried out CPD, and how would you carry out CPD after this interview?

○ How will you carry out CPD in pre-reg training?

○ What are the issues surrounding CPD?

○ What are your thoughts, good and bad, about EPR and CPD?

○ What is CPD and how important is it? Name the four steps. Do you think CPD should be mandatory?

○ Define competence. What does it mean to you?

○ What is competency-based training?

○ How do you monitor and measure your learning?

○ Give an example of when you developed yourself professionally, how you achieved this and what steps you took.

It is important to note that a career in any clinical science involves lifelong development due to the rapid advances which science is making in optimising patient care. Employers will ask you your plans for continuing education so that you can keep abreast of these changes. There are many courses that pharmacists can enrol on to facilitate this. CPPE offers a variety of self-study courses on both clinical and professional topics.

PROFESSIONAL DEVELOPMENT

Try to visualise the CPD cycle when answering these questions.

○ What is CPD? How is it different from CE?

Continuing professional development (CPD) is the means by which members of professional associations maintain, improve and broaden their knowledge and skills and develop the personal qualities required in their professional lives. The CPD cycle comprises four factors:

- *Reflection*
- *Planning*
- *Action*
- *Evaluation*

As pharmacists we need to reflect on our practice. CPD requires us to take personal responsibility for the identification of our learning and development needs and, importantly, for subsequent evaluation of our success in meeting those needs. We are to be the drivers of our learning and development.

Continuing education requires pharmacists to keep our knowledge and skills up to date and addresses new concepts in the delivery of pharmaceutical services, for example, attending courses on certain disease states. Previously, after attending the course and receiving the certificate, there was nothing more for pharmacists to record. Nowadays if they were to attend a course, they would have to reflect upon it and show how this has helped improve their practice.

○ If you were expecting positive feedback from your tutor but instead it was negative, what would you do?

I think it is human nature to be disheartened when first receiving negative feedback. But after careful consideration, one should realise that negative feedback, when justified, will only help to make someone a better pharmacist. I would ask my tutor which particular aspects of my performance were good and which needed more work. After taking the comments on board, I would make a conscious effort to improve on my deficiencies.

○ What do you hope to achieve at the end of your pre-registration year?

In order to become a successful pharmacist, I need to have strong foundations on which I can later build. The first step is to have a successful career as a pharmacy student. The second step is the pre-reg year, where I would like to gain the skills necessary to become not just a competent, but rather an extremely able clinical pharmacist.

○ Do you think it is important to reflect on your work? Why?

I think reflection is an extremely important part of career development. I think that after completing every task, we should always ask ourselves: 'How could I have improved on that?' Individuals who are always satisfied with their work, in my opinion, have less chance of bettering themselves than people who always look to improve. Reflection is an important part of the process of gaining experience.

POLICIES AND PROTOCOLS

○ What is clinical governance?

○ What do you know about the term 'clinical governance'?

○ Clinical governance is an umbrella term: what do you understand about it?

○ Can you tell me how clinical governance will affect you, as a pharmacist, in the future?

○ How would you implement clinical governance in community pharmacy?

○ What is *A Spoonful of Sugar*?

○ Tell us about *A Spoonful of Sugar* and clinical governance.

○ How does the *A Spoonful of Sugar* report affect hospital pharmacy?

○ Do you know what the term 'concordance' means? What factors affect concordance and how can pharmacists play a role in enhancing concordance?

○ Have you come across the document *Pharmacy in the Future?* Can you tell me a few targets that pharmacy departments in the UK need to meet?

○ What is the *Agenda for Change*?

○ Discuss the disadvantages of the *Agenda for Change*.

○ What is the *Clinical Management Plan*?

○ What is the *NHS Plan*?

○ What are your views on the OFT report on community pharmacy?

○ What do you think of the new contract – any positives and negatives?

○ What impact do you think the new contract will have on hospital pharmacy?

○ What have you heard about the government doing to reduce risks?

○ What is a primary care trust (PCT)? How can community pharmacists play a role in this?

○ Do you have any concerns about the hospital trust being a specialist one?

○ What is the FDA?

○ Can you tell me what NICE stands for and what it is?

○ What does NSF stand for? (Make sure you skim-read a NSF so you can talk about it; e.g. if going for Great Ormond Street then skim-read an NSF for paediatrics.)

○ What are your views on supplementary prescribing? How is this different from patient group directions?

○ What do you know about supplementary prescribing?

○ What is meant by the term 'patient group direction'? How is this different from supplementary prescribing?

○ Tell me what you know about pharmacists becoming prescribers.

○ What is medicines management?

○   What is repeat dispensing?

○   What is the function of the RPSGB?

○   What are your views on it, i.e. the professional and regulation roles?

○   What is the difference between POM, P and GSL? Can you give examples of drugs in each category?

○   Define as many abbreviations as possible from a list.

○   What is the future of pharmacy?

○   What are you opinions on robotic dispensaries? What are the advantages and disadvantages of such a system?

○   What are the advantages and disadvantages of e-pharmacy?

○   What are the advantages and disadvantages of e-prescribing?

○   Tell us about electronic recording.

○   What are your views about electronic versions of medical notes?

POLICIES AND PROTOCOLS

○   What is medicines management?

An article I read in the Pharmaceutical Journal stated that 'medicines management explains how pharmacists and other health professionals should get more involved in a new and co-ordinated approach to ensuring patients make the most of their medicines'. This is a new role for pharmacists and it is very exciting for us to be involved with this, since we are the pioneers of medicines.

○   What is the *Agenda for Change*?

Agenda for Change *is a recent initiative in the NHS. It has caused many conflicts! It is a new scheme which governs pay for hospital and primary care pharmacists.*

THE NHS

○   How would you convince someone to give you funding for a new aseptic unit in the hospital?

○   If you wanted to build a chemotherapy unit, how would you convince the trust to invest money in it? What implications would this have? What are the advantages and disadvantages?

○   What is a foundation hospital and what are diagnostic centres?

○   What are the issues surrounding people who visit the UK for 'treatment holidays'?

○   Who is the current health secretary?

○   If you were health secretary for the day, what changes would you make?

○   Do you think government-run health care is better than private health care?

○   Do we complain too much about the state of the NHS?

○   Do you think it is reasonable that hospitals are having to meet harsh demands set by politicians?

○   Can the NHS and private health care work side by side?

○   Give examples of modernisation in the NHS. What are the advantages and disadvantages?

○   How do you see technology developing in the NHS in the future?

○   Can you see the NHS surviving in the future?

The National Health Service (NHS) is a government-owned body that aims to provide each and every British citizen with free/subsidised health care. As a pharmacist, you will either be an employee of the NHS (as in hospital) or you will be given a subsidy for providing an NHS service (community pharmacy). Therefore, it is clear that whichever branch of pharmacy you choose to embark on, you need to have a good insight into the NHS and political issues surrounding it.

The NHS is funded by taxpayers (i.e. the working public), therefore, taxpayers have a right to know where and how their money is being spent within the NHS. As opposed to a privately run health care system, the NHS aims to give patients quality of care whilst maintaining economic efficiency. It is for this very reason that the NHS is constantly in the limelight and under scrutiny. The key phrase here is 'cost–benefit ratio'.

You should have a clear understanding of the structure of the NHS (this is taught in most pharmacy courses). This should provide you with the basic foundation to critique news articles.

You can refer to the following websites to learn more about relevant issues:

- www.nhs.gov.uk
- www.bbc.co.uk/health

THE NHS

Note: Sit on the fence! Try not to criticise the NHS too much, as they are going to be your future employers! If you are asked about your opinion on the NHS, the best approach is to consider some of the points which, in your opinion, would make the NHS a better health care provider; however, do maintain that we are extremely fortunate to have a totally free health care structure. (Hint: study the structure of the Swedish health care system, which is totally free, and very efficient. Compare and contrast a few points between their health care system and ours, and use these when answering such questions to look really slick!)

Always remember that if any new innovative treatment is to be brought into the NHS, it has to have a cost–benefit ratio proven!

○ If you wanted to build a chemotherapy unit, how would you convince the trust to invest money in it?

I would start off by explaining to the trust that the patients who require chemotherapy would probably be referred to tertiary centres which, in some instances, may be strenuous for patients. Chemotherapy is not just about administering medication; it is also about dealing with the psychosocial implications of cancer which can be done efficiently in a chemotherapy unit, especially if this unit is close to home. Furthermore, a local chemotherapy unit will lessen the burden on the tertiary centres, allowing them to deal with more complicated cases. I do understand that everything comes at a cost. However, in my opinion, there is a significant benefit to be achieved from this cost, thus making it a worthwhile investment.

○ Where do you see the NHS in 5 years' time?

It is difficult to give a definite answer to this question as the NHS is being dramatically restructured as we speak. Many factors are making the future of the NHS unpredictable, for example, the restructuring of postgraduate training which doctors receive, the enforcement of the European working time directive which limits the amount of hours health care professionals can work, and the emergence of private independent treatment centres. With so many changes in the melting pot, I think it would be naive of me to give a clear answer of where the NHS will be in 5 years' time. However, I would say that we are very fortunate to have a totally free health care service and it is important that we do what it takes to keep it running efficiently.

THE WORKPLACE

○ What are the negative aspects of community and what are the negative aspects of hospital?

○ What skills do you think a community pharmacist should possess? Which of these skills do you have?

○ What problems do you think community pharmacy is facing?

○ What do you see as the role of the hospital pharmacist?

○ Why did you not choose hospital or industrial pharmacy?

○ Where do you think pharmacy as a profession fits into the health care world?

○ How would you change the role of the pharmacist?

○ How can you as a pharmacist help change the face of pharmacy?

○ How can you as a pharmacist help with the needs of the patient?

○ How do you think you are assessed for competency for the pre-registration year?

○ What will you see as a challenge in your pre-registration year?

○ What do you want to achieve from your pre-registration year?

○ What do you think is the role of the pre-registration co-ordinator?

○ What do you think we are looking for in a prospective pre-reg applicant?

○ What can you bring/offer to our department?

○ What are the competencies pre-reg students have to meet? How would you meet them practically? What would you do if you didn't know them?

○ How would you advertise your products in a pharmacy?

○ How would you increase the sales and business for this company?

○ Talk about a situation where you had to try really hard to sell something to a patient.

○ If you were a store manager and your retail and prescription sales were low, what would you do to increase them?

○ What aspects would you consider if you were opening your own pharmacy?

○ What different types of communication can you have with your patients/customers?

○ If you had a rude and difficult customer, how would you handle him/her?

○ Can you give us a situation during your community placement where a customer was very dissatisfied? How did you deal with it? How did you manage to turn the situation around?

○ When have you turned around a situation from a customer being very angry to being happy?

○ Can you tell us a situation when you felt you provided good service to a customer?

○ Give an example of a situation where you showed business focus in the chemist (or if you haven't any community experience, any other real-life situation).

○ Give an example where you have suggested a change at work. What did you suggest and is it still being acted upon?

○ If it is a busy afternoon, and you are in charge of everything in the dispensary, how would you ensure all the goals were met?

○ If you were unhappy about something in the company you work for, how would you approach the problem? Give examples.

○ How would you conduct a training session for junior recruits?

○ A patient comes into the pharmacy wanting to buy ibuprofen, which his friend recommended. What would you do?

○ How would you feel if a technician managed you?

○ What do you think of the role of a dispensing technician?

○ What is the current role of the technician in hospital pharmacy?

○ If you are in a dispensary with technicians training you a lot of the time, how would you react?

○ What are the advantages of having technician-led dispensaries? Do you think technicians should manage dispensaries?

○ What are your views on ward-based technicians?

○ What is your view on pharmacy technicians?

○ If pharmacy were a blank paper, what would you put in it? Which roles would you employ?

○ What are your views on selling statins over the counter?

○ You're on a ward as a pre-reg student with a pharmacist, the pharmacist is called away and a patient catches your attention before you can follow the pharmacist. The patient explains she is taking a medicine that may be causing diarrhoea and wants advice on the medication. What do you do?

○ Put the following in order of priority that you would handle them, with 1 being first and 4 last. You're a pharmacist in a hospital dispensary at lunch time with two other technicians.

   ● You pick up the phone and a doctor is on the other end wanting advice about a drug that has caused an adverse reaction.
   ● A consultant has appeared at the outpatient hatch and wants to write a prescription for himself.
   ● The technician opens the inpatient hatch and a nurse is waiting for a TTO as a patient's ambulance has arrived.
   ● The other phone rings and there is a patient on the end of the line wanting advice about some medication he was given yesterday to take away.

   Justify each decision.

○ If a patient urgently required medication, it was critical for him to receive it before he left and he was in a real rush, what would you do if there was insufficient supply?

○ Scenario: you have only an hour at the ward: which kind of patient would you prioritise to see first?

○ What would you do if a patient urgently required his medication and you did not have enough of a supply?

○ How would you prioritise the following tasks? What would you do and to whom would you speak regarding this situation? You are assigned a rotational ward round and you have a project deadline on Friday, but the dispensary is busy and they have asked you to help out there during your lunch hour.

○ What would you do if it was a Saturday afternoon and it was just you and an assistant in the dispensary, and a patient was at the hatch, a nurse needed help and the phone was ringing?

○ A drug is urgently required for a patient. The wrong drug arrives to the ward – what do you do?

○ What would you consider urgent tasks and important tasks within a hospital? Give examples.

○ If a pharmacist was complaining to you that she did not like a colleague of yours, what would you say?

○ What would you do if a locum came in drunk?

○ What would you do if your colleagues were underperforming?

○ What would you say to a consultant if he said you were taking over his role and why?

○ What would you say to a colleague, also a pharmacist, who was complaining that a technician was taking over your roles?

○ How do you work with other people to achieve a goal?

○ What measures have you seen in place within the department to reduce risk?

○ What is the role of a pharmacist in managing the risk of drugs on a ward?

○ What can pharmacists do to ensure that medication errors, particularly with other health care professionals, are reduced?

○ How does a pharmacist on ward ensure the safety of medications?

○ How would you react to working in a mental unit?

○ What factors (diseases and practical care) do you have to consider when serving the East London population?

○ What can pharmacists do to help the elderly? Consider that they may have arthritis, poor eyesight and be forgetful.

○ Does the pay in hospital affect you, seeing as you have done experience in community only?

○ Give your opinion on complementary and alternative medicine.

○ If you did a presentation and you only got an acceptable mark, whereas your colleagues got an excellent mark, what would you do?

○   What do you think about competency-based training?

○   How do you assess how well a pharmacy is functioning?

○   Name a change in pharmacy at the moment.

○   What are the issues/developments in pharmacy at the moment? Tell us about the good and bad points.

○   How do you think pharmacy is progressing in terms of technology? Give examples.

○   In your opinion what is the future of pharmacy? Where do you see yourself fitting into that?

○   Where do you see the NHS in the next 5 years?

○   What do you see as the future role of pharmacists? Do you think you will be able to cope with the extended roles?

○   What does the future hold for pharmacy over the next 5 or 10 years?

Questions relating to the workplace are testing your initiative and your ability to think laterally. Common themes focus on prioritisation, work ethics and conflicts at the workplace. These questions may seem aggressive to the student. However, no doubt you will already have been in similar situations, for example in weekend employment or even among your peers.

The best way to prepare for these questions is to brush up on your common sense!

THE WORKPLACE

Note: Some people struggle with these questions, simply because the scenarios put forward are situations which you have probably never encountered before (or so you think!). However, these questions are simply testing your common sense. And if you analyse these questions you will find that you have been in similar situations before, maybe with friends, or perhaps in a Saturday job which has nothing to do with pharmacy.

○   It is a Saturday afternoon with just you and your assistant in the dispensary. A patient is at the hatch, a nurse needs some help and the phone is ringing. How would you handle this situation?

   Note: These questions are very popular, and test your skill of prioritising your work. In the above scenario, your patient is clearly your main priority. However, you have two 'barriers' to the patient – the phone and the nurse! Everybody knows how annoying a ringing phone is, so it would probably be wise to pick up the phone, and take a name and number which you can call back on. Then speak to the nurse, and tell her that you can help her after you have dealt with the patient. If it's urgent, the assistant can make a start on whatever she wants. You now have your path clear for the patient, so give her what she wants! And remember, you have made promises to the nurse and the person on the other end of the phone that you will get back to them, so be sure to do so!

○ What would you say to a consultant if he said you were taking over his role and why?

Note: Any potentially confrontational situation should be dealt with in a private setting. Try to be diplomatic, but at the same time, show that you would maintain your honour as an important member of the team.

These issues are best dealt with in a private setting. Therefore, I would try and meet the consultant in his office. I would ask him why he feels this way. I would acknowledge that his clinical experience is far greater than mine. In fact it is a fruitless exercise to compare each of our clinical exposures. However, being a pharmacist I am also a valuable member of the team looking after the patient. It is important for me to let my views be known to all members of the team. It is not my intention to take over the consultant's role; I am merely giving my opinion. If this seems overzealous, I would apologise and explain that I am passionate about the patients.

○ What would you say to a colleague, also a pharmacist, who was complaining that a technician was taking over your roles?

Note: This is basically the team-dominator question worded differently!

○ How would you explain to a doctor that he has prescribed an incorrect dose for a patient?

Note: Another confrontational setting. The worst thing for doctors is to be humiliated on the ward. They generally have to accept the humiliation if they are getting stick from their seniors. However, they will not appreciate you telling them they are wrong in public! Find a quiet moment, have your evidence at hand to support your viewpoint and discuss the matter diplomatically.

If I noticed this, I would try to find that doctor at a time when he is not busy, and take him to one side to have a private word with him. I would explain to him, as diplomatically as possible, that I felt the dose of drug x that has been prescribed is in my opinion incorrect. I would support my viewpoint with some evidence, maybe from a recent journal article or the BNF. If the doctor acknowledges this, then that is the end of the matter. However, if the doctor feels angry about what I have said, then I would maintain that I am only doing what I feel to be in the patient's best interest. If the doctor continues to be angry, and proceeds with the incorrect dose, then at this point I would try to involve senior members of the team.

GENERAL MISCELLANEOUS

○ Describe yourself as a person.

○ Describe some of your personal qualities that would help you as a future pharmacist.

○ What are your strengths and weaknesses?

○ What is your greatest achievement?

○ What are your bad points?

○ What has been your biggest disappointment?

○ What was your biggest mistake?

○ Explain your strengths and weaknesses. How can you make your weaknesses your strengths?

○ Sum up your strengths in three words.

○ What is your proudest achievement?

○ Tell us a bit about yourself, especially about your Erasmus placement.

○ How would your colleagues describe you?

○ What would your friends say about you if you were not present?

○ How would your friends describe you in three words?

○ What would your family say about you?

○ How would you describe yourself to someone who did not know you?

○ How would you describe yourself to a patient?

- How would your friends describe you as a person and how would your enemies describe you?

- What would a past employer say your weakness is?

- What was the greatest challenge you have ever encountered?

- What areas would you like to improve about yourself?

- What three qualities do you feel you need to improve upon?

- What did you do as head girl?

- How did you handle the transition from school to university?

- How will you tackle the more mundane aspects of the pre-reg year?

- Can you do multitasking? Give an example.

- What skills do you need to develop in the year?

- What skills do you think a pre-reg needs?

- What skills do you think a pharmacist needs?

- What do you think is expected of you this year?

- How do you think you will be assessed this year?

- What are you looking forward to this year?

- What do you think the RPSGB expects from pre-regs?

- How do you think your role will change from the beginning of the year to the end of pre-reg year?

- What three things would you like to achieve by the end of your pre-reg year?

- What do you anticipate as your training needs during the pre-reg year?

- What are your concerns about pre-reg?

- What challenges do you think you will be facing during your pre-reg year?

- What do you think you will enjoy most about pre-reg?

- What appeals to you about hospital pharmacy?

- Why did you choose pharmacy as a career and why community pharmacy?

○ Why would you suggest pharmacy as a career to someone?

○ What qualities do you think a good pharmacist should possess? Which of these qualities do you have?

○ Why pharmacy? And why your chosen school of pharmacy?

○ Why have you chosen hospital pharmacy and why specifically this hospital?

○ Why hospital pharmacy? What qualities do you have that would help in that role?

○ Why have you chosen the hospitals you have applied for?

○ What are your interests?

○ Recreational activities: tell us about them and how do you manage them alongside academic studies?

○ How do you organise your time? How do you divide it?

○ What do you do to relax? How does this help you?

○ What extracurricular activities do you take part in? Have you developed any transferable skills from this?

○ What do you do in your spare time? How do you balance this with your work?

○ What do you feel passionate about?

○ How do you measure your own success?

○ What did you learn about yourself when you were conducting your summer placement in community/hospital/industry?

○ What did you learn at Boots?

○ What have you learnt in your placement?

○ What did you enjoy most in your placement?

○ Tell us about your pharmacy experience and what you learnt.

○ Tell us about your work experience (whether it is pharmacy or not). What did you learn from this? What skills have you developed from your work experience?

○ Tell us about any previous work experience you had. What did you learn and what did you like about it?

○ What pharmacy experience do you have? Discuss.

○ What did you do over the summer (as regards work experience)?

○ Tell us about your work experiences.

○ Tell us about your experience at Guy's and St Thomas' and your audit?

○ How did you cope with meeting new people?

○ When did you see yourself implementing a change? What was that change and how did you implement it?

○ When did you ever overcome a barrier? How did you do this and what was the outcome?

○ When have you had to build relationships with people with whom you are unfamiliar? How did you manage to do this? Could you improve on this?

○ How have you dealt with conflict?

○ When have you been in a situation of conflict? How did you resolve it? Would you do anything differently next time?

○ Give an example of a time when you have inspired somebody.

○ Describe a situation where you used your initiative to solve a problem.

○ Give an example where you had to prioritise your work.

○ Tell me a time when you were very pressurised. How did you deal with it?

○ Give a situation where you had to meet a deadline. How did you meet it?

○ How do you cope with stress?

○ Describe a stressful situation and how you dealt with it.

○ Tell me a time when you have handled a difficult situation well.

○ Tell me when you had to deal with a difficult person.

○ When have you volunteered to do something and it was successful?

○ Can you give a situation when you organised something well?

○ Give an example of an objective and how you worked towards it.

○ Give a situation where you learnt a new skill.

○ Can you give an example where you had to undertake responsibility?

○ Explain a situation where you have shown responsibility.

○ Who is your role model and why?

○ When have you changed your plans for others?

○ What is customer service? How do you give good customer service? Tell us about one time you had to provide good customer service.

○ Give us an example of where you have experienced bad customer service.

○ Give us an example of where you have provided good customer service.

○ What do you understand by communication?

○ How can you use communication in the pharmacy? What forms?

○ Describe a time when you offered good customer service.

○ Give an example when you went that extra mile for a customer.

○ Describe a time when you faced a difficult customer.

○ Describe a time when you delivered customer service using different types of communication.

○ Which do you prefer – lab work or ward work? Why?

○ You had some trouble in your first year: why do you think that is and how did you deal with it? How did it benefit you?

○ I see you invested the time you had during your retake year wisely: tell me what you did. If you had the choice, would you rather fail your first year again knowing that you benefited so much or would you rather not? And would you deal with it differently? If the situation (failing) occurred again, say during you pre-reg, how would you deal with it? What were the lessons you learned?

○ Moving on to the positives, what was your greatest achievement and why?

○ You lived locally from primary school until university, so how can you demonstrate that you can be a responsible and an independent person?

○ Tell me a time you worked on a project (either as a team or by yourself). What went well? What went badly? What would you improve next time?

○ What does quality mean to you?

○ Give me an example when you were led by someone.

○ Tell me about a time when you led people.

○ Give an example when you made a decision that upset others around you.

○ What would you do if you were expecting positive feedback from your tutor and instead it was negative?

○ If you were doing a project, what would you do from start to finish?

○ Describe a time when you failed to meet a deadline.

○ What qualities should a successful pharmacist possess?

○ Tell me about competence.

○ What do you think is lacking in your placement?

○ How do you organise your workload?

○ How would you plan a project from start to finish?

○ What is the difference in the law of dispensing in Malaysia, where you did some work experience, compared to in the UK?

○ Do you think it is right to dispense medicine without the pharmacist on site?

○ What made you decide to go for hospital pharmacy, especially as you have extensive community experience?

○ What qualities should a good pharmacist possess?

○ Why do you think pharmacists should have to be pre-reg co-ordinators when they don't receive any extra pay for doing so?

○ Why do we take pre-registration students when we are not obliged to? What do we get for doing this when it costs us so much?

○ What are competencies?

○ What is competency-based training?

○ Have you been to the RPSGB?

○ What can you offer this hospital trust?

○ What can we expect from you?

○   What can you give us? What do you have to offer?

○   Why do you think we should employ you?

○   Why do you want to work with us?

○   Why did you choose London, this area and this hospital?

○   Are you willing to work long hours? 50 hours a week, Monday to Friday?

○   Why should we pick you out of all the applicants we are interviewing?

○   Why have you applied to our drug company in particular?

○   Why do you want to be in industry?

○   What did you get to do in community pharmacy?

○   Why have you chosen our hospital?

○   What are our company values?

○   What personal qualities do you think this hospital is looking for?

○   Why did you rank us third in your choice of hospital?

○   Which hospital would you choose at UCL?

○   Which other hospitals did you apply to and why?

○   Have you been offered interviews with any other hospitals?

○   Did you expect to hear from us for interview?

○   Have you got any other interviews?

○   Is there anything you want to ask us?

These are generic questions that one would expect in any interview and can be a good starting point for an interview, for example, discussing why you chose pharmacy as a career.

This section also contains some difficult questions, some of which have a controversial slant to them.

A good approach to answering any question with a controversial theme is to 'sit on the fence'. Here follows a generic example:

Do you think we have too many immigrants in this country?

This question may seem very hostile when initially considered. However, using the above approach it can be tackled with ease. On the one hand you could discuss the benefits of this issue (e.g. allowing individuals to better themselves) and then on the other hand consider the problems associated with it (e.g. burden on taxpayers).

When asked such general questions, try to draw in examples from non-pharmacy settings. This will give the interviewer a better insight to you as a person and demonstrate your multidimensional personality.

Although many of these questions seem basic, if you answer tactfully, you can impress interviewers and your responses may single you out from the rest of the candidates.

GENERAL MISCELLANEOUS

These are your general 'run-of-the-mill' questions that you would probably be asked in any interview situation. Everyone tends to give very similar answers to these questions, so try to stand out from the rest by being innovative!

On the issue of being different, one example springs to mind. A student applying to study at a renowned university was asked to write an essay defining courage. While all his fellow students were scribbling away, he wrote an essay which was one sentence long. He headed the page as follows:

Courage
This is courage....

He got a place to study politics, and came out with a first-class degree.

○ What would your fellow peers say about you?
   Note: A simple enough question – this is your opportunity to tell your potential employers how good you really are! However, if you do choose to balance out all the praise with some criticism, always use examples that could easily be turned into strengths. It's probably best to let them ask you your pitfalls as opposed to you volunteering them.

○ What is the greatest challenge that you have encountered?

One of the greatest challenges I have ever had to face is to turn down a slice of double-chocolate cheesecake whilst on holiday when I was suffering from traveller's diarrhoea!

This answer may seem totally ridiculous! Most people will probably say that their greatest challenge was something academic, or perhaps something sport-related. The above answer is totally different from the norm, and shows that you have the courage to say something like this in a stressful setting, and that you have a sense of humour. It also shows the interviewers that you have an interest in travel, and it may spark them to ask about your travelling experiences – now that's so much easier than talking about the side-effects of rifampicin!

○ What are your strengths and weaknesses and how can you make your weaknesses your strengths?

Note: Try to be selective in your choice of weakness here. It's probably best not to say 'My biggest weakness is that I'm lazy!' One of the biggest clichés of this question is 'My biggest weakness is that I'm a pedantic perfectionist'. Although the perfectionist example is tried and tested, try to find a weakness like that which you could easily turn into a strength.

One of my biggest weaknesses is that I'm a bit of a chatterbox. Sometimes this can be good, as it keeps people cheerful, but some people may find it a little annoying at times! I suppose I can turn this weakness into a strength by limiting the amount I talk, just to the level where it's friendly banter at work, which will help to keep the morale of my team up!

○ Describe a situation where you used your initiative to solve a problem.

Note: Wide range of examples! Here's one:

Every Saturday, I used to work at an estate agents office showing properties to potential buyers. I was on my way to a property viewing when I noticed that one of the tyres on my car had a puncture. I pulled up at the side of the road, and put on my hazard lights. I then phoned the potential purchasers of the property to let them know of my misfortune, and that I would have to cancel the viewing, and suggested calling the office to rearrange. As I proceeded to change the tyre things went from bad to worse, as when I checked the spare tyre, it also happened to be flat! Now a fully booked diary on a Saturday without a car is impossible. I then rang the manager at the office to let him know of the situation, at which point he called the emergency tyre service. They had my car fixed within half an hour, and the rest of the day ran smoothly.

This answer is a good example, as the interviewee has given a scenario where she tried her level best to deal with the situation, before seeking the help of her seniors.

And finally

I hope that you have found the material in this book useful.

It cannot be overemphasised how important it is to be prepared for the entire application and interview process.

As mentioned previously, competition is high and vacancies are limited, so try your hardest and eventually the hard work will pay off.

I would like to end by summarising some key points regarding the pre-registration application process:

- Apply everywhere for pre-registration
- Apply all over the UK
- Spend time on your application forms
- Prepare well before the interview
- Attempt to answer all questions in the question bank
- Be confident on the day
- Be yourself

Good luck once again and keep up the good work!

Appendix 1

Pre-registration recruitment guidelines from the RPSGB

> The following information has been taken from the RPSGB website: *Preregistration recruitment letter December 2006.* www.rpsgb.org/pdfs/preregrecruitguid07.pdf (date of access 6 March 2007). Guidance does change and it is therefore very important that you always refer to the latest guidance. Please see the Registration and Support section of the RPSGB website for latest information (www.rpsgb.org).

PREREGISTRATION RECRUITMENT[1]

As you may already be aware, the RPSGB produces a set of guidelines outlining the Council's view of the best practice for the recruitment of pharmacy students into preregistration training posts as outlined in the RPSGB Undergraduate Bulletin For 3rd Year Pharmacy Students.

In recent years, organisations have commenced the recruiting process earlier and earlier, and this has caused concern for students who have been asked to give a formal acceptance to an offer before having the opportunity to attend interviews with other organisations.

After discussion between RPSGB and Senior Executives of pharmacy employers it was decided that in 2007 employers may hold interviews and make formal offers at their convenience. If the student is happy with the offer they can accept the position *at any* stage. Employers expect that acceptance or refusal of a position must be received by **Friday 5th October 2007 (NB the date will change from year to year, check this on the Society's website)** and students should not be pressured to give a formal acceptance prior to this date. **Pressure to make decisions is neither in the employer's nor the employee's best interests.**

As in accordance with the RPSGB Code of Ethics, it would be considered unethical to accept a job offer in any way (including a verbal acceptance) and then to later retract it.

This system is in place to enable you to hold one offer while waiting for interviews with other employers. It is not intended to enable you to hold on to several offers at once. If students do hold on to offers that they are not going to accept on 5th October, then it prevents the employers offering those places to other students who may really want them. Those students may then have to accept a post they don't really want for fear of being unemployed. This is not in anyone's best interests, and certainly not students'. If you are not going to accept a post, please let the employer know as soon as possible.

It is hoped that this will result in a more orderly recruiting system for all parties involved and allow students to make informed decisions that they can adhere to. If you are being pressured or are aware of anybody pressuring students to give a formal acceptance prior to the 5th October, please contact the Preregistration Division at the RPSGB on 0207 572 2372 or email Prereg@rpsgb.org.

The following Guidelines outline the RPSGB Council's view of the best practice for the recruitment of pharmacy students into preregistration training posts. Employers who comply with these Guidelines will expect students applying to do likewise.

Students Best Practice Guidelines are that they will:

- Properly research opportunities and organisations and concentrate on those organisations in which they have a genuine interest when making applications.
- Be prompt, courteous and honest in all dealings with employers and notify them immediately if they decide not to proceed with their applications at any stage.
- Be honest with employers about the preferred aspect of practice for preregistration training, other applications made or existing offers of preregistration employment.
- When attending interviews at employer's premises, seek only repayment of reasonable expenses incurred.
- Only accept offers of employment if conditions are acceptable and ensure that terms of employment are provided in writing.
- Once an offer has been accepted in writing, decline all other offers and inform all other potential employers to whom they have applied that they have made a commitment elsewhere.
- Clearly state at the time of acceptance if they wish to qualify their acceptance in any way (the possibility of further study represents such

a qualification) and recognise that such qualification may affect the terms of the offer.

- Recognise that both the offer of a post and its acceptance form a contract unless conditions are attached to either and that written acceptance must be honoured other than in the most exceptional circumstances i.e. those which are beyond their control or which they could justify as being professionally acceptable.

Employers **Best Practice Guidelines are that they will:**

- Make available material to give students an objective picture of their organisations and to provide information about specific preregistration training opportunities.
- Offer equality of opportunity and avoid in their literature or application forms for employment in the UK any reference that might be construed as unfair discrimination.
- Acknowledge receipt of all applications and inform students whether or not they are to be invited for interview.
- Students should not be pressured to give a formal acceptance to an offer prior to the date set by the RPSGB.
- Notify the result of an interview promptly to a student.
- When requesting a verbal, provisional response immediately or very soon after the interview, give a time allowance of not less than 3 days for students to respond formally in writing to a written offer and recognise that it is the written acceptance, which is binding. (This is to avoid the use of unreasonable time-scales which can limit the ability of students to make informed decisions, prejudice the recruitment activities of other employers and give students cause to accept offers and renege on them later.)
- When students have other possibilities to consider, inform them if the offer can be held open and for how long.
- Not give an impression that any commitment to work after the preregistration period is enforceable in law.
- Make clear to applicants whether and what expenses will be paid for attendance at interviews.
- Agree referees with the candidate and not seek reference from a person not so designated without the candidate's agreement.
- Indicate clearly to the candidate and to the referee whether or not the offer is conditional on the reference.
- Explain clearly the terms and conditions of service in offer letters and state whether or not an offer is conditional on degree classification, medical examination etc.

- Recognise that both the offer of a post and its acceptance form a contract unless conditions are attached to either make clear to the applicant that an offer of employment is subject to the Royal Pharmaceutical Society approving the programme of training and/or the premises and/or the tutor when such is the case.

This appendix has been reproduced with permission from the Royal Pharmaceutical Society of Great Britain.

Reference

1   Preregistration recruitment letter December 2006. www.rpsgb.org/pdfs/preregrecruitguid07.pdf (date of access 6 March 2007).

Appendix 2

Example CVs and covering letters

Name: SD •
Address: 32 Flower St
Dollis Hill
London
Tel: 09654 3456
E-mail: SD@hotmail.com

Sex: Male
Date of birth: 11/03/1984
Marital status: Single
Nationality: British

Education

2003–Present (Graduate July '07)	**London School of Pharmacy** Masters of Pharmacy (MPharm)
2001–2003 A levels	**Islamic College for Advanced Studies (ICAS)** Chemistry (A), Biology (C), Computing (C)
1997–2001 GCSEs	**Gayton High School** 11 subjects, all ranging from A to C grades

Work experience

July '06 — **Barts and the London NHS Trust**
- Understand the nature of hospital pharmacist
- The use of robots in pharmacy

June '06 — **St George's Hospital**
Went on a number of different wards, gaining confidence in approaching elective patients to confirm information such as medical history

Jan–Feb '06 — **Manichem Great Holland Pharmacy**
- Emergency cover provisions
- Treatment policies and fee collection
- A greater understanding of how a private pharmacy works

Aug–Sep '05 — **Al Sundos Pharmacy (Dubai)**
- As all of normal community pharmacy

	but a flavour of pharmacy work in a different country with different requirements
June '04	**Lloyds Pharmacy (Virginia Waters) + Lloyds Pharmacy (Hounslow)** • Structure and nature of the pharmacy • Premises and facilities • Support services and suppliers
Feb–Mar '03	**Willesden Surgery** • Understanding the duties and responsibilities of the medical team • Joint clinics, combining different specialties to manage patients with head and neck injuries • Communicating and informing patients of various outcomes
Jun–Jul '02	**Marylebone Medical Centre** • Patient reviews post surgical investigation • Pain management of psychological origin • Patient referrals to other specialties

Skills

- Excellent knowledge of operating systems, including Windows XP, 2000 and NT
- Great time management and organisation skills
- Great knowledge of general laboratory work
- Excellent communication and customer communication skills
- Also excellent in Microsoft Office software suite, including Word, PowerPoint and Excel. Proficient with the internet and online research
- Effective team-player, with ability to provide essential interaction and participation

Interests and activities

- I am an amateur photographer with special interests in stills and portraits pictures. I undertook self-directed learning to further my knowledge and techniques in photography. I am currently learning about digital picture editing.
- I thoroughly enjoy travelling as it has allowed me to understand and experience different cultures. I recently travelled to Dubai, United Arab Emirates and Bahrain. I was able to travel around these countries and have the opportunity to speak to the locals to gain a better understanding of their history and culture. I used my photographic skills to capture some of the great scenic views and local people.

Referees available on request

CV

Name: HP
Date of birth: 10/09/1983
Address: 153 Acacia Grove, Wembley
Contact number: 078123 6548

Qualifications

GCSEs
Arabic A*, Mathematics (pure + applied) B, Science Double Award BB, Art B, Graphics Design B, Geography C, English Language C, English Literature C.

A levels
Physics B, Chemistry B, Mathematics C

Other
Computer literature qualification, driving licence

Current status
Pharmacy student at London School of Pharmacy, year 3
Topics covered: biotechnology, sterile products, biochemistry, microbiology, oncology, pharmaceutics, pharmacy practice and therapeutics, pharmacology, chemistry and toxicology

Work history

CNE Computers: sales assistant, 1998–1999
I gained a great deal of insight into one of my subjects of interest, computers. This was my first job and I was able to relate to customers' needs and demands and I took on responsibilities. Naturally I gained a great deal of computer knowledge.

ANK Electronics: sales adviser/assistant, 1999–2000
I met a wide range of people from different backgrounds and this helped me improve my communication skills. I also assumed various responsibilities which helped to make me overall a more responsible person.

Elite Marketing: group leader, 2001–2002
I worked as a sales promoter in what is called affinity marketing. This was my first opportunity to take full responsibility and demonstrate my communication and selling skills, as the pay was performance-based. I also worked in telemarketing and trained new recruits.

Blockbuster Entertainment, central London: duty manager, assistant manager 2002–2004
I was promoted from sales assistant to duty manager in 2 months, and then to assistant store manager. I enjoyed working in busy conditions and organising a team for customer services. I was also given great responsibility in managing and training other staff.

Bush Pharmacy: dispenser, patient advisor, summer 2005
I had been eager to try out community pharmacy and I was grateful for this opportunity. I worked here for 2 weeks, gaining a great deal of experience, and I became proficient in dispensing and pharmacy practice under supervision. I was able to communicate with and relate to patients and work with them to reach a goal. This was a valuable time when I got a taste of what could be an everyday activity for me.

Prince Pharmacy: patient adviser and sales assistant, summer 2005
Continuing in pharmacy, I worked in Edgware Road, London, for about a month where I was able to speak to Arabic customers and meet their needs. The pharmacy did not dispense NHS prescriptions so the main focus was pharmacy (P) and over-the-counter medications. I gained a good deal of knowledge of the business and management of the retail sector in pharmacy.

Statement
I am a well-skilled communicator on my way to getting a Masters degree in pharmacy. I have worked in various companies and have gained management and people skills, as well as marketing and advertising skills in the retail sector. I also have a good knowledge of computer hardware and software and great time management skills. I'm also a very good group leader and problem-solver and make decisions for which I take responsibility, and I am always cheerful. I have a mechanical mind that's always expanding on how things work and why. I'm hoping for a job in the health sector that will further my ambition of having a great role to play in drug development and health care in my future career.

Interests
I'm a very social person with a good sense of humour and I love to get out often. I enjoy movies, and I play sports, mainly swimming, netball and badminton. I also very much enjoy repairing and fixing mechanical objects, which requires both patience and determination, and I have a great interest in politics and international affairs.

References
Available on request

NK

Address (home)
161 Arsenal Road
Littleman
Derby
DE23

Nationality British
Date of birth 19-09-83
Marital status Single
Gender Female

Telephone +44 (0) 1332 545 675
+44 (0) 7970 123456 mobile

E-mail NK@hotmail.com

Academic history
March 2005–July 2005
University of Southern California–Los Angeles
- Three months' extramural placement carrying out my final-year dissertation and project write-up
- Carrying out a drug delivery project in the Pharmaceutical Sciences department. I carried a project titled *Correlation between Conformation and Transduction of Cationic Peptides*, which entailed working in detail with heparin and four different peptides, in the laboratory and using computer-based modelling programs
- Furthering my knowledge in this field and being able to organise my time academically and socially and being able to enhance my communication skills to work with others

Oct 01–present
University of London, School of Pharmacy
- MPharm degree

Sept 98–May 01
Derby Tertiary College Wilmorton
- A levels: Chemistry (B), Biology (B), Mathematics (C)

Sept 93–Jun 98
Littleover Community School, Derby
- GCSEs: 10 subjects (grades A*–C), including Mathematics, English and Double Science Award

Work experience/employment
August 2005–present
Manor Pharmacy
- Dispensing medicines
- Shadowing pharmacists
- Serving customers

July 2005
Derbyshire Hospitals: Derbyshire Royal Infirmary and Derby City General
- Two-week pharmacy placement
- Shadowed pharmacists, technicians and consultants
- Gained an insight into the role pharmacists play in hospitals
- I managed to build on my communication skills with other health professionals and learnt how to communicate with ill patients in a hospital environment, to give them exactly the care they needed
- The experience highlighted the significance of a multidisciplinary team working together

June 04–Sept 04
GlaxoSmithKline (GSK)
- Rotated between Clinical Trial Supplies, Clinical Manufacturing, Pharmaceutical Development and Marketing
- This was my second insight into how the pharmaceutical industry operates, but this time on a larger scale
- Having followed protocols, I worked with new compounds and tested them for their properties and prepared them for future testing in New Chemical Entities
- I was given the opportunity to work on the team for Macleans, Lucozade and Sensodyne brands. This gave me insight into how the products were marketed to the public from adverts on the television to pharmacy in-store posters
- In the manufacturing suite I observed how tablets and capsules for clinical trials were formulated; this was very enjoyable as I have a keen interest in this part of drug development
- Thanks to GSK, I had a solid introduction to the pharmaceutical industry. I discovered the different responsibilities that would be expected from me as a future employee in big pharma. I understood that it is crucial to be a good team-player

June 03–Sept 03
Polytherics Group, School of Pharmacy
- Research assistant
- Learning to research literature using websites, databases and scientific journals

Oct 02–Dec 02
Boots the Chemist
- Trainee health care assistant
- Sales assistant
- Stock control-ordering
- Cashier
- Experience gained in working as a team and in a business environment

Responsibilities
June 2005–Present
The School of Pharmacy, University of London Students' Union
- Student's Union **Entertainments Officer**
- Third year running in the university's union
- Organising entertainment events for the university and being involved in the organisation of events for the University of London Union
- Liaising with the current president on issues involving all types of entertainment
- Being delegated specific tasks and managing them with the help of other union members
- Potential events being organised are the annual freshers' boat party, the annual mid-season ball, the Christmas party and the introduction of the new students

October 2004–Present
The School of Pharmacy, University of London Students' Union
- Students' Union **Executive Board Member**
- Sitting in on meetings and overseeing any difficulties the current presidents were having
- Being able to contribute my ideas and the knowledge I gained as joint-president
- A lifelong commitment

October 2004–Present
The School of Pharmacy, University of London basketball team
- Official school team **Coach**
- Playing in national tournaments and achieving satisfactory results
- Organising weekly practices and meetings
- Organising fortnightly games against other universities around the country
- I learned to further my skills in organising my time academically and for the university and built the reputation of the team. I have been loyal to the team and helped achieve high standards, prioritising my time so that neither the team nor my studies were affected
- I have listened to other players' opinions of how to achieve better results.

June 2003–June 2004
The School Of Pharmacy, University of London Students' Union
- Students' Union Joint **President**
- Co-ordinating freshers' week, Christmas, Easter and end-of-term events/sixth-form leaver parties
- Organising paper work
- Handling students' money
- Advert and poster design work
- Designing the Students' Union magazine

- I learnt how to work with others to achieve great results within the team
- I worked as part of a 10-member team delegating tasks with my co-president, making sure the tasks were carried out on time and to a very high standard
- I gained valued experience as a team leader in how to be diplomatic and considerate to others

Additional qualifications/skills
- NHS Community Dental Nursing (evening class)
- RSA computer literacy and information technology (CLAIT) level 4 (computer literacy)
- Full clean driver's licence
- Excellent interpersonal and communication skills
- Advanced skills in organisation, prioritisation and working under pressure to meet deadlines

Interests and hobbies
- Reading fiction books
- Travelling: South Asia, Europe and North America
- Keen interest in sports: basketball* (member of the Derby Storm under-21 team), netball*, volleyball*, hockey*, tennis and badminton, coaching the School of Pharmacy basketball team
- Keen interest in martial arts, including, tae kwon-do and wing chun kung fu*
- Cooking oriental and Asian food
- An avid interest in music: I am becoming a disc jockey in my spare time

*taught or captained.

References

MK

161 Rykneld Road
Littlover
Derby
DE23
Tel: +44 (0) 7970 711234

29 July 2006

Dear Mr PS

Re: Pharmacy Pre-registration Application

I am writing with regard to a pre-registration position within your firm. I enclose my curriculum vitae for your review.

I have recently completed my third year in Pharmacy and am applying for a pre-registration training programme for 2007 within industry.

I am determined to work in the industry sector of the pharmaceutical profession and I am very keen to obtain my crucial training to develop and strengthen myself for this career path. As such I see the position being offered within your company as key.

Working for you would give me a solid introduction into industry pharmacy. A lifelong ambition to work for Pfizer, the leading UK pharmaceutical company, would be fulfilled. Working for another well-known company has enhanced my drive in pursuing a career in the pharmaceutical industry and would enable me to make an immediate contribution to the company.

I see myself as dynamic, vibrant and innovative, all of which have led to me tackling and overcoming new challenges. I am very determined to be successful and to do what I do to the best of my ability.

I have held many positions of responsibility which have developed a number of my interpersonal skills, such as leadership, communication and the ability to encourage and motivate team members. I have demonstrated that I can work effectively whether as part of a team or individually not only at work, but also in both sport and academia. This has helped me to build good relationships with both work colleagues and customers/patients.

I feel that my experience and skill set, combined with my motivation and confidence, will help me to become a valuable asset to your firm. I relish the chance of joining Pfizer and hope to do so with great enthusiasm.

If you require any additional information from me at this stage, please do not hesitate to contact me.

I look forward to hearing from you.

Yours sincerely

MK

My name is HS. I am a 22-year-old Pharmacy student at University of London's School of Pharmacy. I am in the third year of the MPharm course and nearing the end of the first semester.

I am keen to obtain a pharmacy placement on the summer placement programme run by the hospital. I feel it is vital to gain pharmacy experience in a hospital environment before I reach my pre-registration year. It would also be a good opportunity to be part of the health care team and work as a group, in contrast to the individual settings seen in community pharmacy.

In summer 2006 I undertook a summer placement at two different community pharmacies, Bush and Prince Pharmacies, for around 6 weeks. These pharmacies had different approaches. In Bush Pharmacy I was involved in the whole dispensing process which the pharmacist monitored, whereas at Prince Pharmacy I was more of a sales person as the pharmacy did not have an NHS contract and only dispensed private prescriptions. Most of the work involved meeting customer demands and giving advice on P and over-the-counter medications. My work also involved stock and order management, prescription management, operating tills, cashing up, attending to customer services and regular shop work. I thoroughly enjoyed the experience.

I have enclosed a copy of my CV.

Thank you.

Index